Pure-Tone
Audiometry and Masking

Core Clinical Concepts in Audiology

Series Editors
James W. Hall, III, Ph.D.
Virginia Ramachandran, Au.D.

Pure-Tone Audiometry and Masking
by Maureen Valente, Ph.D.

Pure-Tone Audiometry and Masking

Maureen Valente

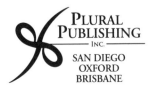

PLURAL
PUBLISHING
INC.

SAN DIEGO
OXFORD
BRISBANE

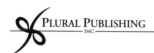

5521 Ruffin Road
San Diego, CA 92123

e-mail: info@pluralpublishing.com
Web site: http://www.pluralpublishing.com

49 Bath Street
Abingdon, Oxfordshire OX14 1EA
United Kingdom

FSC
Mixed Sources
Product group from well-managed
forests and other controlled sources

Cert no. SW-COC-002283
www.fsc.org
© 1996 Forest Stewardship Council

Library of Congress Cataloging-in-Publication Data

Valente, Maureen.
  Pure-tone audiometry and masking / Maureen Valente.
      p. ; cm. — (Core clinical concepts in audiology)
  Includes bibliographical references and index.
  ISBN-13: 978-1-59756-340-6 (alk. paper)
  ISBN-10: 1-59756-340-4 (alk. paper)
  1. Audiometry. I. Title. II. Series.
  [DNLM: 1. Audiometry, Pure-Tone. 2. Hearing Disorders—diagnosis. 3. Perceptual
Masking. WV 272 V154p 2008]
  RF294.V35 2008
  617.8'9—dc22

                                                          2008049456

Contents

Foreword

How can we make learning in audiology more effective? This is the question that we began with in the design of the Core Clinical Concepts in Audiology series. Our answer is revealed in the construction of the books of the series. Herein we seek to provide palatable and useful information to students and practitioners to develop and refine clinical skills for audiology practice.

By and large, texts available for our field provide exhaustive examination of broad topic areas. Although these texts are useful and necessary for advanced scholarship, we currently lack pedagogic materials that focus on basic clinical methods and knowledge. The books in this series are designed for teaching and learning.

These books are written for the student. The scope of practice for audiology has expanded dramatically since the inception of our field. Today's students must acquire a tremendous arsenal of clinical skills and knowledge in a very short period of time. The books of the CCC series are meant to be clear and comprehensible to students, focusing on the content necessary to achieve knowledge and skills for clinical practice. Furthermore, the books are designed to be economical, both financially and in time spent in learning.

These books are written for the clinician. With expansion of the scope of audiology practice, currently practicing clinicians must acquire new skill sets while continuing to serve their patients. Not a small feat. Hard-working practitioners deserve educational materials compatible with the real-world demands of fast paced and time-limited clinical practice. In response to these needs, the books of the

CCC series are designed to be concise. The succinct construction of the series is meant to allow readers to efficiently acquire the essential concepts and skills described in the books.

These books are written for the instructor. Most instructors of audiology courses are familiar with the frustration of searching for materials that cover the topics which reflect the learning outcomes of their courses. Especially lacking are materials designed to promote clinical learning. The books of the CCC series are designed to focus on specific areas of clinical practice. They are targeted toward the learning outcomes commonly found in audiology curricula. Due to the economical nature of the books, instructors can feel comfortable in creatively combining different Core Concepts in Audiology books to support the unique and diverse learning demands of specific courses.

These books are written for the user. The needs of the reader are our primary concern. These books are written with the purpose of helping readers learn to be outstanding clinical audiologists. To be sure, these are lofty goals. The authors of the CCC series books have put forth their best effort to accomplish these goals.

Pure-Tone Audiometry and Masking by Maureen Valente serves as the cornerstone for the Basic Audiometry component of the CCC series. Dr. Valente's extensive and successful experience in teaching students of audiology provides an ideal foundation for authorship of this title. This book covers the most fundamental and important skill set that audiologists will acquire. Covering everything from acoustics, psychoacoustic methods of obtaining threshold, procedures for air- and bone-conduction testing, masking, testing of special populations, to identification audiometry, the text is comprehensive in nature. Chapter 9 of the text utilizes numerous case examples to provide readers with a context for in-depth learning of material and serves as a bridge to thinking in terms of clinical practice. The organization and construction of the book works to achieve the goals of the CCC series, providing information in a manner consistent with the needs of readers. We believe that this text will provide the reader with a foundation of knowledge to implement and improve clinical skills in pure-tone audiometry and masking and that this book will be instrumental in the development of fundamental clinical audiologic skills.

James W. Hall, III, Ph.D.
Virginia Ramachandran, Au.D.

Preface

The Core Clinical Concepts Series is designed to present a series of textbooks, each of which addresses a topic in an in-depth and comprehensive manner. *Pure-Tone Audiometry and Masking* serves as one of the first in the series, helping to provide building blocks toward the basic comprehensive audiologic evaluation. Because pure-tone audiometry historically has served as an important foundation for patient evaluation, material contained allows the audiologist to build toward more sophisticated measures.

Prior to learning protocols of clinical audiology, a strong scientific base is necessary. Following Introductory information in Chapter 1, an Acoustics Overview is provided in Chapter 2. Simple Harmonic Motion (SHM) is discussed, along with elementary properties of sound: frequency, intensity, and temporal aspects. Although SHM and pure tones are extremely relevant when evaluating hearing, the patient deals with speech stimuli within everyday listening environments. Because speech is composed of numerous frequencies and intensities, study of complex waveforms is included.

As the examiner prepares for pure-tone testing, he or she must become familiar with equipment, calibration procedures, and daily listening check protocols. Chapter 3 describes these processes, in addition to other aspects of patient preparation and infection control. Threshold, or the softest level of intensity at which a patient responds, has been extensively studied in both hearing science and clinical audiology literature. Various methods for ascertaining threshold are discussed in Chapter 4, leading into study of the audiogram form, audiometric symbols, and crucial elements of air and bone conduction testing. Variables that may affect audiometric test results are presented, in addition to methods for controlling for such variability and obtaining the most accurate results possible.

Once beginning clinicians have mastered threshold measurement and other clinical procedures, they proceed to master one of the most important aspects of all: interpretation of test findings. Chapter 5 is centered about audiogram interpretation and critical parameters of determining type, configuration, magnitude, and symmetry. This chapter concludes with suggestions for explaining audiometric findings to the patient and family.

Clinical masking, discussed in Chapter 6, is one of the most difficult areas for the audiologist to employ. It is crucial, however, to prevent participation of the nontest ear during testing. This chapter includes explanation of masking theory, rules of when to mask, formulae for determining masking levels, description of the actual procedure, and examples of difficult cases. Many patients may not be evaluated through utilization of conventional audiometric techniques. Information provided in Chapter 7 includes evaluation of the pediatric patient, from a brief overview of electrophysiologic measures to discussion of unconventional behavioral techniques. This is followed by discussion of tuning fork tests that may help with interpretation of findings and evaluation of hearing impairment. Further sections include evaluation of nonorganic hearing loss and uses of ultrahigh-frequency audiometry.

Hearing screening may be efficiently performed with large groups of potential patients, to determine those who require thorough audiologic evaluation. This procedure may also be performed as an integral component of a speech, language, or other type of evaluation. Information contained in Chapter 8 provides guidelines for pure-tone screening across the life span. Within Chapter 9, the reader may gain practice with sample audiograms that may be noted with frequently seen conductive, sensorineural, and central disorders.

In concluding Chapter 10, pure-tone audiometry is summarized from past, present, and future perspectives. Clinical pearls and pitfalls are discussed as related to patient preparation for testing and the actual performance of pure-tone audiometry and masking. Insights toward test outcomes and report writing are provided, along with additional uses of pure-tone stimuli within a diagnostic audiology practice. Integration of pure-tone audiometry and masking with other components of audiology's scope of practice is presented as a critical component.

The student encounters a number of difficult concepts early on during an audiology program, including decibel references, calibration of equipment, audiogram interpretation, and masking. The reader is encouraged to utilize this textbook to fortify knowledge related to these and other concepts and to strengthen performance of pure-tone audiometry and masking. Once a comfort level is reached regarding equipment and protocols, the audiologist is well on his or her way toward becoming a professional who is adept at interpretation and exercising sound clinical insights. May knowledge gained here serve as a foundation for building and for enhancing learning toward these and additional audiologic diagnostic measures.

Acknowledgments

I was honored to receive the invitation from Plural Publishing to write this textbook, which serves to combine two of my greatest professional passions: writing and working with students. To paraphrase a popular political slogan, it takes a professional community to construct such a work of educational material. I am deeply grateful to the Department of Speech and Hearing Sciences at the University of Illinois in Champaign-Urbana for providing me with such an excellent undergraduate and graduate foundation for clinical practice. Furthermore, my past clinical and teaching experiences, including at St. Louis University, have served to strengthen my knowledge base so that I may share it with others. I would also like to thank the Program in Audiology and Communication Sciences (PACS) at Washington University in St. Louis on several levels. The Washington University faculty provided exceptional mentoring throughout my doctoral studies, contributing significantly toward my becoming a better academician.

It has been a pleasure to have served as PACS' Director of Audiology Studies since August of 2005. I wish to thank Dr. Bill Clark, Ms. Beth Elliott, Ms. René Miller, and Ms. Beth Fisher within PACS' Administrative Team for support and assistance during this period and especially during the writing of this textbook. As a strong student advocate, I would like to express deep gratitude to current students and to those who have touched my life over the past 20 years.

Above all, I would like to thank my family for boundless love, devotion, and support, both professionally and on a personal level.

Thank you so much, Mike, Michelle, and Anne, for all that you do and for all that you have meant to me. Finally, this textbook is dedicated to the memory of my parents, Maurice and Lora Kennedy. They taught me the immeasurable value of reading, learning, and education long before I was able to even speak these words.

About the Author

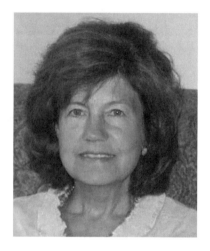

Maureen Valente, Ph.D., earned her Bachelor of Science and Master of Science degrees in Speech and Hearing Science from the University of Illinois in Champaign-Urbana. She spent her Clinical Fellowship Year in the Chicago area, in the office of G. E. Shambaugh, M.D. Subsequent work experiences included private practice and medical settings in the Kansas City and Omaha areas, including employment at Boys Town National Research Hospital in Omaha.

After moving to the St. Louis area, Dr. Valente was employed as a full-time faculty member for 18 years within St. Louis University's Department of Communication Sciences and Disorders. She graduated with her Doctor of Philosophy degree in Speech and Hearing Sciences from Washington University in St. Louis. Shortly thereafter, she was delighted to accept a position as the Director of Audiology Studies within the Program in Audiology and Communication Sciences (PACS) at Washington University School of Medicine. She carries a joint appointment within PACS and as an Assistant Professor within the university's Department of Otolaryngology. Areas of interest include development of Au.D. education, diagnostic audiology, auditory processing disorders, and vestibular evaluation across the life span.

1 *Introduction*

Pure-tone audiometry serves as the foundation for comprehensive audiologic evaluation, typically performed during the first patient visit and also during subsequent visits, when indicated. Its roots date back to the 19th century, although the procedure as we know it today was first described by Bunch and Dean in a 1919 presentation to the American Otologic Society (Bunch, 1943). One of the first vacuum tube audiometers became available in the United States by the early 1920s; over the past 90 years, the profession has seen computerization of equipment and miniaturization of parts. Pure-tone and other audiometric procedures gained popularity post-World War II when the audiology profession arose from a fine blending of disciplines: rehabilitation, psychology, medicine, speech-language pathology, and others.

Most individuals are familiar with audiometry's very basic premise of "raising a hand when one hears a tone," although procedures and their interpretations are actually much more complex. During testing, the skilled audiologist presents calibrated stimuli to the listener, via evidence-based procedures, and carefully records patient responses. As one views the spectrum of a pure tone, one notes frequency across the abscissa from low to high and amplitude along the ordinate, from softer to louder as the graph moves upward. A pure tone spectrally represents that extremely narrow band of the center frequency, with a designated amplitude as well as rapid signal rise and fall times. Spectrally, the pure tone is differentiated from speech stimuli, in that the latter are composed of numerous frequencies and numerous amplitudes as a function of frequency.

Specialized and often computerized equipment is utilized within a sound-treated booth, in order to perform pure-tone testing. In addition to learning detailed procedures for conducting pure-tone testing, the audiologist must ensure that he or she implements techniques most appropriate for the individual patient and that valid/reliable test results are obtained. The beginning audiology student progresses from learning to manipulate equipment dials to recording responses on the audiogram. As the student develops from technician to insightful clinician, he or she acquires further competency related to interpretation of results. Finally, insightful recommendations toward remediation are made following interpretation.

RATIONALE FOR PURE-TONE AUDIOMETRY

Pure-tone audiometry is one of the first steps in diagnostic work with a patient who has sought audiologic services. The patient listens for tones that are presented via assorted types of earphones and other transducers and the audiologist records threshold, or softest level heard, in each ear for each of the various tones. Although these tones are usually continuous in nature, pulsed and/or frequency-modulated tones may be used in certain clinical situations. In preparation for performing pure-tone audiometry, the audiologist must learn fundamentals of acoustics in order to understand basic parameters of stimuli presented: primarily frequency, intensity, and temporal dimensions. Although humans typically listen to speech stimuli in their everyday listening environments, it is important to also gain information about responses to tonal stimuli. The comparison of speech audiometry and pure-tone findings may help ensure test reliability, as these measures should be in close agreement with one another. Tonal and speech audiometry will also provide the clinician with complementary information, specifically regarding how the patient is responding to simple sound waveforms and how the patient is responding to more complex waveforms. The audiologist compares unaided and aided results to the speech spectrum or "speech banana" that may be superimposed upon the audiogram form. Through these results, the audiologist may estimate audibility of average conversational speech for the patient. Furthermore, he or she may determine which particular environmental and speech sounds may be heard by the patient and which are inaudible.

Upon entering the clinical setting, the clinician is fortified with detailed information regarding audiometric equipment, equipment calibration, proper equipment usage, patient preparation, and thorough pure-tone testing procedures. One of the most important aspects of performing pure-tone audiometry with a patient is audiogram interpretation. Once thresholds are obtained and the symbols are generated on the audiogram form, the audiologist prepares for one of the most important responsibilities of all: application of clinical insight. Through interpretation, he or she determines information about four very important test parameters: magnitude, type, configuration, and symmetry of hearing impairment. From the audiogram, the audiologist may determine if a hearing loss is present, whether it is in one ear or both, and the severity of the loss. The audiologist may determine the type of hearing loss and gain insights as to whether the disorder occurs in the middle ear, inner ear, or both areas. Myriad additional diagnostic measures may be in order. The audiologist is also well educated to determine signs and symptoms of patient disorders that occur in the central auditory nervous system and to make referrals to other hearing health care team members, when indicated. Basic audiologic evaluation described above may provide information about symmetry between the two ears and whether sensitivity of one ear is significantly different from that of the other. Finally, the audiologist determines configuration, or shape, of the hearing loss. For example, some patients may hear all tonal frequencies equally. Others may hear lower frequencies better than they may hear higher frequencies, and still others may hear higher frequencies better than lower ones.

PURPOSES

Pure-tone audiometry is a springboard for many other tests that the audiologist may wish to perform. During the comprehensive initial evaluation, the patient typically also undergoes speech audiometry and immittance audiometry measures, in addition to pure-tone testing. The audiologist is well educated regarding hearing disorders and the audiogram types and configurations that accompany these disorders. Once the pure-tone audiogram and accompanying tests described above are completed, the audiologist counsels the patient regarding results and may relay myriad recommendations for treatment. These may include referring the patient for medical or surgical management, scheduling the patient for a hearing aid evaluation, recommending electrophysiologic or other diagnostic measures, determining cochlear implant candidacy, communication strategy training, and a host of many other remediation strategies. The pure-tone audiogram plays a major role in subsequent audiologic recommendations following its completion and in initial steps toward thorough team management of the patient. Pure-tone testing may also be performed as a baseline and in serial fashion, in order to monitor course of a disorder or effects of a toxic agent upon hearing.

There are numerous difficult concepts for a student of audiology to immediately master. These concepts include calibration of audiometric equipment according to standards of the American National Standards Institute (ANSI) and interpretation of the audiogram. In addition, clinical masking is a very challenging concept for the beginning clinician to understand and implement in a clinical setting. This phenomenon involves introducing a noise to the non test ear under certain circumstances, so that the non test ear does not participate in evaluation of the test ear during pure-tone audiometry. If the masking procedure is not implemented correctly, serious consequences may occur, such as misinterpretation of hearing loss type or underestimating magnitude. Upon inaccurate audiogram interpretation, errors will follow regarding course of remediation recommended for the patient. These and other challenging concepts are studied in depth as one learns proper pure-tone audiometric techniques, with detailed study of clinical masking serving as an integral aspect of attaining valid results and true thresholds during pure-tone audiometry.

SCOPE OF PRACTICE ISSUES

The profession of audiology has transitioned to a doctoral profession over the recent two decades, such that a doctoral degree is the entry-level degree. As one examines the many audiologic test procedures being performed within numerous clinical settings, it is important to keep in mind scope of practice issues. Pure-tone audiometry must be performed by a clinician who has an earned degree in audiology and who is licensed within the practicing state. In some settings, audiometric technicians may perform pure-tone diagnostic measures following extensive training and under an audiologist's supervision.

In contrast to diagnostic evaluations, pure-tone hearing screenings are quick and efficient procedures utilized with large groups of individuals to determine those who must be referred for a thorough diagnostic evaluation. Through use of a hearing screening, the examiner determines if hearing is within or below normal limits, as opposed to ascertaining exact hearing levels. Furthermore, type of hearing loss may not be determined from a screening. These screenings may be performed by a speech-language pathologist or other support personnel, as long as supervision by an audiologist is present (ASHA, 1997). A hearing screening is also an integral component of a speech-language evaluation, to rule out contribution of hearing loss to a speech and/or language disorder.

REFERENCES

American Speech-Language-Hearing Association. (1997). *Guidelines for audiologic screening.* Rockville, MD: Author.

Bunch, C. C. (1943). *Clinical audiometry.* St. Louis, MO: C. V. Mosby.

2 *Acoustics Overview*

SIMPLE HARMONIC MOTION

A natural sequence for students of Audiology is to acquire knowledge related to basic hearing science concepts. One of the primary areas is principles of acoustics, including properties of sound and how those are clinically applicable to audiometric testing procedures (Berg, 2004; Daniloff, Schuckers, & Feth, 1980; Denes & Pinson, 1973; Durrant & Lovrinic, 1995; Gelfand, 1990; Gerber, 1974; Gulick, 1971; Hamill & Price, 2008; Haughton, 2002; Yost, 2000).

As a sound waveform travels through a medium, molecules are displaced and alternately formulate highly dense areas of compression and less dense areas of rarefaction. The most common medium is air and the pressure variations travel through this medium toward the receiver or listener. The most basic form of sound is called Simple Harmonic Motion (SHM) and may be visually represented as a simple sine wave. In Figure 2–1, such a simple sine waveform is shown with time across the *x*-axis and amplitude or magnitude of molecule displacement along the *y*-axis (courtesy of Barry Truax, Simon Fraser University). The compressions may be noted by highest peaks in an upward direction and the rarefactions by lowest peaks in a downward direction. Following the completion of one compression and one rarefaction, one cycle is completed and another begins, at least in such a periodic or replicable waveform.

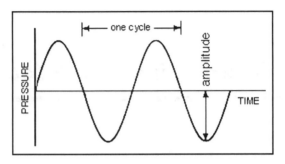

Figure 2–1. Simple harmonic motion. (Courtesy of Barry Truax, Simon Fraser University, www.sfu.ca/sonic-studio/handbook/Sine_Wave.html)

FREQUENCY

The first parameter of sound, frequency, is defined as the number of cycles completed within one second (Yost, 2000). Frequency is measured in hertz (Hz), referring to the number of cycles occurring per second, and frequency differences are perceived by the listener as changes in pitch. The greater the number of cycles present in one second, the higher the pitch perceived by the listener.

The average normal human listener typically hears a frequency range from approximately 20 Hz to 20 kHz (Gerber, 1974). When one views audiometric equipment and an audiogram as shown in Figure 2-2, one observes that patient hearing is routinely evaluated from 250 Hz through 8000 Hz. The six major audiometric frequencies are shown across the top of the graph: 250, 500, 1000 (1k), 2000 (2k), 4000 (4k), and 8000 (8k) Hz. These frequencies occur at octave intervals and the audiologist also learns rules for testing mid-octave frequencies of 750, 1500, 3000 (3k), and 6000 (6k) Hz.

Standardized audiometric procedures include measuring threshold at the above described test frequencies, instead of the entire fre-

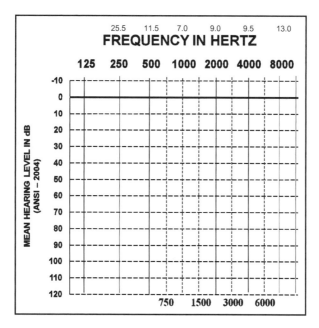

Figure 2–2. Audiogram showing audiometric zero and corresponding RETSPL levels as a function of frequency.

quency range of human hearing, for a number of reasons. Because the most critical frequencies for perception of speech stimuli are within the range of 250 to 8000 Hz, it is important to test this range. Testing of the entire frequency range of human hearing would be too time and labor intensive with little additional clinical benefit.

Simple harmonic motion may be represented visually as a sine wave and is heard as a pure-tone stimulus. Two of the very few examples of SHM within our environment are sounds emitted by vibrating tuning forks, sometimes utilized during medical evaluation, and pure tones emitted by clinical audiometers during pure-tone testing. When one views audiometric equipment, he or she notes that the frequency dial is one of the major controls. The audiologist manipulates this control in order to deliver signals of various frequencies during pure-tone testing. Upon ascertaining threshold, results are recorded on the audiogram; the x-axis shows "Frequency in Hz" from lower frequencies (125 or 250 Hz) on the left side to higher frequencies (8 kHz) on the right side, as noted in Figure 2–2.

INTENSITY

The second parameter of sound is amplitude or intensity, measured in decibels or dB. Changes in amplitude are perceived by the listener as changes in loudness and are represented on the sine waveform as differences in y-axis height. The decibel scale is such that 10 dB increments grow logarithmically; thus, the pressure increase from 20 to 30 dB is 10 times greater than the increase from 10 to 20 dB and this phenomenon continues in ratio form as one moves up the scale. The decibel scale is a relative one, indicating that there may be negative values represented, and a value of 0 dB does not mean "absence of" sound. Patients may very well exhibit thresholds of 0 dB HL or even −10 dB HL. The decibel may also be viewed as a ratio, where some form of varied and measured output is compared to a reference value that remains constant. Most audiometers test from −10 dB HL, representing a very soft sound, to a very loud sound of 110 dB HL or greater. Intensity limits of the equipment will vary, depending on frequency tested and on audiometer type.

Understanding the decibel and its varying references may present challenges to the beginning audiologist. There are four major decibel references, some of which are used more in diagnostic audiology than others. When the clinician refers to "dB," it is important to label with the appropriate reference.

Just as there is a typical frequency range for normal human listeners, one may also describe a "dynamic range" (DR) of intensity and this DR varies from individual to individual. DR is defined as ranging from threshold, the very softest sound a listener may hear, to the Loudness Discomfort Level (LDL), or the loudest comfortable sound. This is an important clinical concept and represents the range of residual or usable hearing available to the listener. Furthermore, this is the range that the audiologist and patient have available for application of auditory rehabilitative strategies.

dB IL (Intensity Level)

This is a power measurement where an output in watts/cm^2 is measured and compared to a constant or reference. This constant value is analogous to threshold, or softest sound heard by average normally hearing listeners. Professionals may see this decibel reference in hearing science and engineering applications, but do not utilize it often in clinical audiology. The formula for obtaining dB IL = $10 \times \log$ Io/Ir where Io refers to the varied intensity output in watts/cm^2 and Ir refers to the intensity reference that is also expressed in watts/cm^2.

dB SPL (Sound Pressure Level)

This is a pressure measurement where an output in dynes/cm^2 is measured and compared to a constant or reference. As with dB IL, this constant value is analogous to the softest sound heard by average normally hearing listeners. The formula for obtaining dB SPL = $20 \times \log$ Po/Pr where Po refers to the varied pressure output in dynes and Pr refers to the pressure reference that is also expressed in dynes. Although audiologists do not often make calculations utilizing these formulae during a typical workday, understanding of underlying theory is crucial.

Applications utilizing dB SPL are many within the realm of clinical audiology. For example, audiologists working in industrial settings may utilize sound pressure level meters (SPLM) to make noise measurements within the work environment. Similarly, audiologists working within a school setting who are interested in classroom acoustics may utilize a SPLM for making ambient noise measurements in various types of classroom environments. While reporting the noise levels in these examples, the audiologist reports "X dB SPL" of noise occurring within that environment. A final application example relates to electroacoustic analysis of hearing aids and other amplification systems, in addition to real-ear probe microphone measures. As specialized equipment generates gain and output curves, the audiologist may observe that maximum output at a certain frequency is "X dB" or that there is a certain amount of gain in dB at another specific frequency. These values are expressed in dB SPL.

dB HL (Hearing Level or Hearing Threshold Level)

Another major control of the audiometer, besides the frequency dial, is the dB dial or intensity attenuator. This dB reference, relating to the audiometer and audiogram form, corresponds to dB HL. In congruence with audiometric results obtained with a piece of audiometric equipment, the audiogram also depicts dB HL along the y-axis, progressing from softer levels at the top to louder levels toward the bottom. The reference for dB HL is "audiometric zero," representing the average human threshold at each individual frequency tested. The description of "audiometric zero" as an average threshold value helps to explain how there is presence of sound at 0 dB HL; thresholds of some normal listeners are more sensitive than this value whereas thresholds of others are less sensitive.

In studying auditory physiology and the ear's response to sound, the clinician learns that the ear is nonlinear (Yost, 2000). The ear demonstrates varying sensitivity, depending on frequency of the stimulus. Specifically, the ear is most sensitive between 1 to 3 kHz and it requires a lesser degree of sound pressure to reach threshold at these frequencies than at lower and higher frequencies. When one views the American National Standards Institute's Specifications for Audiometers (ANSI S3.6, 2004) one may see corrections called Reference Equivalent Threshold Sound Pressure Levels (RETSPLs). These corrections, for use with earphones and similar transducers, are discussed in Chapter 3 describing calibration of audiometric equipment. They serve, however, to help illustrate important differences between dB HL and dB SPL. RETSPL correction values are added to a dB HL reading of the audiometer, in order to convert to dB SPL and to measure these values from a sound pressure level meter. An example of these RETSPL correction values may be seen at the top of the audiogram in Figure 2–2. They serve to illustrate the nonlinearity of the ear concept, demonstrating that it takes less sound pressure at the middle frequency range to reach threshold (in dB HL) or "audiometric zero" than it does in lower and higher frequencies. One may easily see, because of the nonlinearity, that audiometric testing would be very difficult to record and interpret if the audiogram were formulated in dB SPL.

Examples of the dB HL reference in diagnostic audiology are straightforward. Simply, results obtained via an audiometer and/or recorded on a standard audiogram are in dB HL. For example, if a threshold obtained for the right ear at 2 kHz is 30 dB, it is actually 30 dB HL. If the audiologist measures a Loudness Discomfort Level (LDL) at 105 dB via an audiometer's transducer, this value is recorded as 105 dB HL. Other measures besides pure-tone results may also be reported in dB HL, such as a Speech Recognition Threshold (SRT) or presentation level while obtaining a Word Recognition Score (WRS).

dB SL (Sensation Level)

The final dB type discussed is "Sensation Level" with the reference varying from individual to individual, depending on his or her own threshold. Audiologists learn and implement various diagnostic protocols, with some being threshold measures and others being suprathreshold measures. A simple definition of dB SL is a comparison of an above-threshold presentation level to the patient's threshold. For example, one very common test protocol is to obtain Word Recognition Scores (WRS) at +30 or +40 dB SL so that the patient may receive optimum speech cues possible at such an intensity level. The reference must always be provided when using "dB SL" and in this case it is the person's Speech Recognition Threshold (SRT). With Patient A who demonstrates an SRT of 5 dB HL, the test protocol dictates obtaining a WRS at +40 dB SL (re: SRT) or at 45 dB HL. With Patient B who demonstrates an SRT of 35 dB HL, the test protocol still dictates obtaining the WRS at +40 dB SL (re: SRT), but the presentation level will be different than with patient A. With Patient B, the audiologist will be presenting the stimuli at 75 dB HL. These cases provide further examples of dB HL reference usage and additional applications of dB SL usage may be seen via exploration of other test protocols. Below is another example, with a test protocol that may be performed at +5 dB SL. This time, the reference is the patient's pure-tone threshold at that particular frequency, because the protocol dictates utilizing pure tones, instead of speech, as stimuli during that particular test procedure:

	Pure-Tone Threshold	Protocol: Perform at +5 dB SL	Presentation Level
Patient A	25 dB HL		30 dB HL
Patient B	70 dB HL		75 dB HL

PHASE

Although not represented on the audiogram, phase also is an important dimension for describing characteristics of sound. Phase refers to timing or temporal aspects. If describing one sinusoid, as shown in Figure 2–1, one may refer to phase angle. The sinusoid is compared to 360 degrees of a circle, where the starting point in time tradition-ally represents 0 degrees; the maximum compression represents 90 degrees; the baseline crossing the x-axis between compression and rarefaction represents 180 degrees and the maximum rarefaction represents 270 degrees. Continuous numbers are represented at vary-ing sections of the graph until 360 degrees are reached, at which time the cycle is repetitive. Sinusoids may begin later in time than the one demonstrated. When two or more sinusoids are compared, a phase difference measurement may be observed that compares rel-ative time dimensions of the waveforms. These waveforms may be in phase, where they reach 90 degrees and all subsequent temporal landmarks at the same time and in synchrony with one another. They also may be out of phase, where they reach compressions and rarefactions at different times. Such waveforms may be out of phase by as little as one degree or by as many degrees as exist on the above described 360-degree continuum. Temporal aspect of sound applica-tion in clinical audiology includes understanding of inner ear physiol-ogy, speech perception theories, hearing aid selection and verification strategies, and evaluation of auditory processing disorders.

COMPLEX WAVEFORMS

It is important to discuss Simple Harmonic Motion and its proper-ties, in leading to discussion of pure-tone audiometry. Most signals in our environment, though, are of a more complex nature. Although this textbook focuses on pure-tone testing, these results typically do not stand alone and are accompanied by other very important mea-sures within the battery that utilize speech stimuli. Speech stimuli are excellent examples of complex waveforms that are composed of many integrated and simple sinusoidal waveforms. This integration may represent many different frequencies and many different inten-sities as a function of frequency. Just as a complex stimulus is made up of many sinusoids of varying frequency and intensity, such a complex signal may also be broken down into its individual frequency and intensity components via specialized equipment. Complex signals may take on many forms, with some common examples being vowels of speech that are periodic; unvoiced consonant sounds that are aperiodic; and noise that may be present in the environment. Complex signals may be emitted by audiometric equipment, such as speech stimuli presented via Compact Disk or noise for use in clinical masking and other aspects of testing.

REFERENCES

American National Standards Institute. (2004). *Specifications for audiometers (S3.6-2004)*. New York: Acoustical Society of America.

Berg, R. E. (2004). *The physics of sound* (3rd ed.). San Francisco: Benjamin Cummings.

Daniloff, R., Schuckers, G., & Feth, L. (1980). *The physiology of speech and hearing: An introduction*. Englewood Cliffs, NJ: Prentice-Hall.

Denes, P. B., & Pinson, E. N. (1973). *The speech chain* (2nd ed.). New York: New Anchor Press/Doubleday.

Durrant, J. D., & Lovrinic, J. H. (1995). *Bases of hearing science* (3rd ed.). Baltimore: Williams and Wilkins.

Gelfand, S. A. (1990). *Hearing: An introduction to psychological and physiological acoustics* (2nd ed.). New York: Marcel Dekker.

Gerber, S. E. (1974). *Introductory hearing science: Physical and psychological concepts*. Philadelphia: W. B. Saunders.

Gulick, W. L. (1971). *Hearing: Physiology and psychophysics*. New York: Oxford University Press.

Hamill, T. A., & Price L. L. (2008). *The hearing sciences*. San Diego, CA: Plural.

Haughton, P. (2002). *Acoustics for audiologists*. San Diego, CA: Academic Press.

Yost, W. A. (2000). *Fundamentals of hearing: an introduction* (4th ed.). San Diego, CA: Academic Press.

3 *Preparation for Pure-Tone Testing*

THE HEARING CLINIC

There are many settings where an audiologist may practice and establish his or her hearing clinic. Professional settings include, but are not limited to, private practice, university clinics, medical schools, hospitals, medical offices, school district diagnostic centers, and others. All have capabilities, of course, for pure-tone testing as this is the cornerstone of the comprehensive audiologic evaluation. Varying additional audiologic services may be offered, depending on the type of setting and audiologist area of expertise. Considerations in developing the clinical space include acquiring state-of-the-art equipment, establishing services to be offered, determining types of third party payment accepted, insuring patient accessibility and comfort, maximizing referral sources, and marketing of services.

EQUIPMENT

Pure-tone and other forms of audiometric testing are performed in a sound-treated booth or suite. Booths may be of various sizes and dimensions; larger ones may be required, for example, with pediatric testing and hearing aid evaluation. ANSI (2004) Specifications for Audiometers provide requirements for maximum permissible ambient noise levels within the sound suite, as a function of one-third octave frequency band. These levels are provided under ears-covered with insert or earphone conditions and under ears-uncovered conditions for bone conduction and sound field testing. Although it is a misperception that audiologists test within completely "sound-proof booths," ambient noise must be attenuated sufficiently so that accurate thresholds and other measures may be obtained. The booths may be single- or double-walled to adhere to these specifications. Typically, the suite is situated in a quiet area that will house its weight and where electrical and other interferences may be minimized. The patient is seated within the sound booth and in window view of the examiner, who is seated at audiometric controls outside of the booth when conventional techniques are utilized. Some clinics may house side-by-side booths, with one for the patient and one for the examiner, just as they may house multiple booths for multiple, simultaneous testing sessions. Figure 3–1 shows a sound-treated booth with the audiologist seated at controls of the audiometer while testing a patient, who is seated within the suite.

Audiometer Types

There are five main audiometer types (ANSI, 2004), ranging from Type 1 to Type 5. The lower the audiometer type number, the greater the number of controls and the more sophisticated the capabilities for obtainable measures. Most hearing clinics are equipped with a Type 1 two-channel diagnostic audiometer that has capability for pure-tone testing, speech audiometry, narrow band and speech noise emission for clinical masking, and sound field testing. Portable audiometers are discussed in a later section related to hearing screening, for example, within a school or senior center setting. These pieces of equipment also have applications for bedside evaluation with inpatients. Specialized audiometers are available for automatic audiometry, speech audiometry and ultrahigh-frequency audiometry.

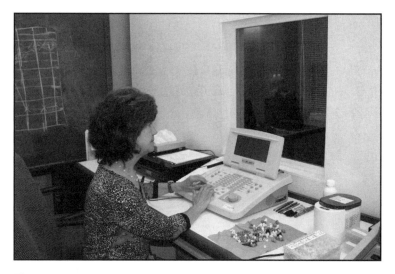

Figure 3–1. Audiologist at audiometer controls engaging in pure-tone audiometry.

Figure 3–2 shows a Type 1 two-channel diagnostic audiometer. As the beginning student is learning the controls, this piece of equipment may be thought of as two simpler portable units placed side by side.

Audiometer Controls

Two major controls, the frequency dial and the intensity (attenuator) dial, are integral components of the audiometer. Although audiometers vary depending on type and function, most frequency dials are capable of emitting signals from at least 125 Hz through 8 kHz. The major discrete audiometric frequencies are included on the dial, as are mid-octave frequencies. There are ultrahigh-frequency audiometers that are portable in nature and are capable of emitting pure-tone signals through 18 or 20 kHz. Some audiometers are capable

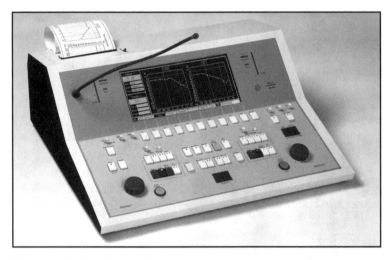

Figure 3–2. Two-channel diagnostic audiometer (with permission from Interacoustics).

of producing signals of both standard audiometric frequency and ultrahigh-frequency.

The frequency dial may indicate a setting for "speech," in addition to the various settings for pure-tones. Speech stimuli may be presented in a live voice fashion by activation of the "microphone" setting. Speech is a complex signal, encompassing many different frequency components and intensities as a function of frequency. This is one reason why both pure-tone testing and speech audiometry are performed with a patient and why the results complement one another. A patient may demonstrate hearing sensitivity within normal limits for reception of speech, while demonstrating a hearing loss at some test frequencies. A patient also may demonstrate poorer speech audiometric findings than pure-tone testing indicates, a "red flag" for possible central pathology or phonemic regression. Conversely, better than anticipated speech audiometric findings may be a sign of nonorganic hearing loss.

The intensity dial also may vary, depending on audiometer type, but many are capable of testing at intensities as low as −10 dB HL. The loudest signal emitted may be as intense as 110 dB HL, although extended range audiometers may emit signals as loud as 125 dB HL. Maximum output in dB HL will also vary as a function of frequency. Although most intensity dials are marked in 5 dB steps, and most testing techniques implement these increments, many audiometers may incorporate steps as small as 1 dB.

The audiologist learns to manipulate the output controls, determining if a signal should be delivered to the right ear, left ear, or both ears simultaneously. The output selector may also help deliver the signal via a choice of many transducers: circumaural earphones, supra-aural earphones, insert earphones, bone conduction oscillator, or loudspeaker of the sound suite. These transducers are plugged into a jack panel located within the sound suite, while corresponding output controls lead from the audiometer to a jack panel located on the outside of the sound suite. When one wishes to present a signal, for example during pure-tone testing, the interruptor switch is used. This control, when "continuously off" and then manually depressed, allows the audiologist to present and control presentation of the stimulus, usually for 1 to 2 seconds during routine pure-tone testing. When the interruptor switch is "continuously on," the tone or other stimulus presented is continuous.

The audiologist also manipulates additional controls called stimulus controls, depending on the type of testing performed. With pure-tone testing, the audiologist selects "tone" as the stimulus, but he or she may also elect to deliver live speech stimuli via the microphone, speech stimuli via the CD player, or various types of noise for masking purposes. These types of noise include narrow band noise, speech noise, and white noise. During pure-tone testing, the audiologist also may choose to present a frequency-modulated (FM) tone or a pulsed tone, depending on the testing situation. Examples of such situations are when a tinnitus patient is unable to discern the pure-tone from the tinnitus or when presenting signals within the sound field system, as might be accomplished during pediatric testing or hearing aid evaluation.

Other types of equipment may interface with the audiometer, for facilitation of testing and recording results. Most audiometers are interfaced with a CD player for use in speech audiometry, auditory processing evaluation, and other diagnostic measures. State-of-the-art technology also allows display, save, and print functions for audiometric data. It is also important for the audiologist to have access to a talk-back system for communication with the patient. The patient, situated within the booth, has access to a microphone that conveys responses and also allows him or her to converse with the audiologist. It is necessary for the audiologist, seated at the audiometer outside of the sound suite, to hear patient responses, and to talk to the patient to instruct and provide reinforcement. Figure 3–3 shows a portable audiometer with major controls demonstrated, including supra-aural earphones and bone conduction oscillator.

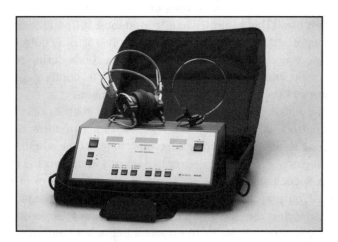

Figure 3–3. Portable audiometer showing major controls (with permission from Maico Diagnostics).

Transducers

Transducers convert one form of energy to another (Decker, 1990; Frank & Rosen, 2007) and are utilized for delivering stimuli during diagnostic testing. All discussed here convert the audiometer's electrical output to acoustical energy except the bone conduction vibrator or oscillator, which makes a conversion to mechanical energy. Earphones are marked in red for testing the right ear and in blue for testing the left ear. All transducers are calibrated for use with a specific audiometer. For this reason, caution must be exercised when switching earphones, or other transducers, from one piece of equipment to another. Supra-aural earphones are embedded in cushions that attach to a headband. The most common types are Telephonics Dynamic Headphone (TDH) 39, 49, and 50 and are illustrated in Figure 3–4.

Occasionally, the audiologist may utilize circumaural earphones, similar to the supra-aural type, with the earphones mounted in plastic domes that completely surround the ear. These types of earphones are commonly seen with industrial testing, testing environments that exhibit higher ambient noise levels, and testing of higher frequencies above 8 kHz. Insert earphones have gained popularity over recent years and a common type, the ER-3A, (Killion, 1984) may be seen in Figure 3–5. The audiologist must select one of three different sizes that is most appropriate for the patient and must insert the foam tips correctly. Specifically, tips must be inserted well into the ear canal, as opposed to only the orifice of the ear canal, and one must allow time for foam tip expansion prior to testing. Insert earphones alleviate testing artifact that may result from improperly collapsing ear canals. Although not a true pathology, collapsed external ear canals may occur from pressure exerted by more standard supra-aural earphones and the inserts ensure a greater degree of canal patency. When the collapse inadvertently occurs, a pseudoconductive hearing loss may be seen on the audiogram and this has implications

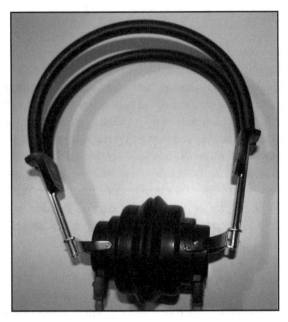

Figure 3–4. TDH 50 P supra-aural earphones.

toward interpretation, medical referral and other forms of patient management. Interaural attenuation (IA) is a term related to the attenuation of a signal as it crosses from the test to nontest ear, leading to the need for clinical masking so that accurate test results may be obtained. This IA value is increased when insert earphones, as opposed to more conventional earphones, are used. That is, participation of the nontest ear is less likely and the need for masking is diminished.

During audiometric testing, signals may also be presented through the loudspeakers that are located within the sound booth, often mounted on or near walls. There may be two or more loudspeakers, with each requiring a wide-frequency bandwidth and smooth frequency response. In addition, they should function in

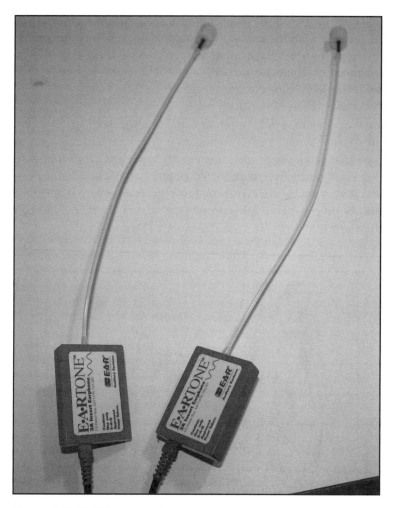

Figure 3–5. EAR insert receivers.

conjunction with the audiometer's intensity capabilities in dB HL. The audiologist may utilize loudspeakers during pediatric testing, for example, when a child may not accept earphones, although the obtaining of individualized ear information is optimum and will not be possible with speaker use. Although real-ear probe microphone systems now exist for hearing aid verification, there also may be instances of obtaining unaided and aided thresholds and other audiometric measures within the sound field.

Presentation of signals through supra-aural earphones, circumaural earphones, insert earphones, and loudspeakers are all examples of air conduction (AC) testing. As one reviews basic anatomy of the ear as related to AC presentation of these signals, one may note that signals are delivered through the outer ear, middle ear, inner ear, and then through the central auditory nervous system (CANS) for further processing. In other words, the signal is delivered through the entire auditory system, as illustrated in Figure 3–6.

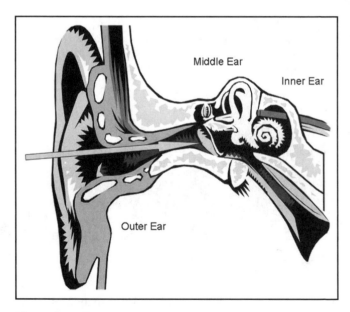

Figure 3–6. The air conduction pathway.

Figure 3-7 shows an audiologist preparing to place earphones on the ears of a patient, in preparation for AC testing. With earphone placement, the clinician must ensure that the earphone diaphragm is directly placed over the ear canal opening.

Bone conduction vibrators are encased in plastic, display a flat circular area for placing on the mastoid (or forehead), and are mounted on a headband. They are present in various sizes, shapes, and weights, with one of the most common in this country being a Radioear B-71 model. Figures 3-8A and 3-8B display figures of this commonly utilized bone conduction vibrator and its placement on the mastoid process of a patient.

These transducers exhibit limitations when coupled to diagnostic audiometers for testing. Because of such equipment limitation,

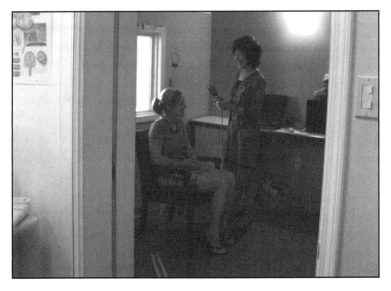

Figure 3–7. Audiologist preparing for air conduction testing with a patient.

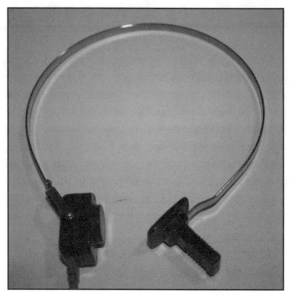

A

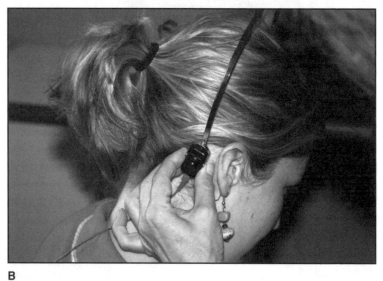

B

Figure 3–8. A. Bone conduction oscillator and headband and **B.** bone conduction oscillator placement on a patient.

clinicians typically are unable to perform bone conduction testing above 4 kHz; also, intensity limits for bone conducted stimuli at test frequencies are lower than they are for air-conducted stimuli and vary according to frequency. In placement of the bone vibrator on the mastoid for testing, the audiologist must make certain that hair is not interfering or that the vibrator is not touching the pinna. The audiologist must be alert for slippage throughout the testing session and must physically change the transducer from the right to left side, as opposed to merely pushing a button to change signal delivery from right to left. As one observes delivery of bone conduction (BC) signals in relation to anatomy of the ear, one notes major differences from delivery of the AC signal. As the signal is delivered through the mastoid bone, it bypasses the outer and middle ear, collectively referred to as the conductive mechanism. The BC pathway is illustrated in Figure 3–9.

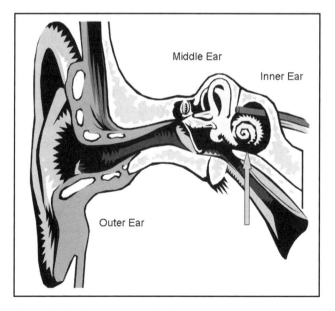

Figure 3–9. The bone conduction pathway.

The signal is delivered directly to the cochlea of the inner ear and stimulates both cochleas simultaneously. Because both cochleas are housed within the bones of the same skull, they are both stimulated when pressure variations set the skull into a vibratory pattern. It is critically important for the audiologist to understand differences between AC and BC signal delivery, as these differences play a major role in determining type of hearing loss and subsequently in determining site of lesion. Similarly, the concept of stimulating both cochleas simultaneously has implications toward clinical masking, as the examiner presents noise to the nontest ear so that accurate tonal results may be obtained in the test ear.

CALIBRATION AND THE ANSI STANDARDS

Just as it is extremely important for the audiologist to demonstrate thorough working knowledge of audiometric equipment and its usage, it is also important to ensure that the audiometer is properly calibrated and in excellent working order. The audiologist should feel comfortable with calibration procedures, should be familiar with ANSI Specifications for Audiometers (2004), and should check calibration according to ANSI required time lines. The relevance of calibration cannot be overestimated. This procedure ensures, for example, that a 1000-Hz tone is actually presented when that is the frequency dial reading. Proper calibration also ensures the clinician that intensity levels delivered are actually as indicated on the intensity dial readings. Standardized calibration allows results from one patient to be compared from clinic to clinic or from visit to visit within the same clinical facility. The procedure also facilitates comparison of results from patient to patient. There are endless possible consequences if patients are tested and results determined with audiometric equipment that is out of calibration. Although the reader is referred to the ANSI Standards (2004) for thorough description of calibration specifications, basic procedures for checking output (intensity) and frequency are described in the following pages.

As the audiologist prepares to check output calibration, major pieces of equipment needed are: sound pressure level meter (SPLM), pistonphone, 6-cc coupler and 2-cc coupler, artificial ear, artificial mastoid, and pressure/free-field microphones. The audiologist measures output with all transducers previously described, utilizing the appropriate coupler and/or microphone. The example provided here is with a TDH-49 supra-aural earphone, with output levels checked one earphone at a time. In preparing equipment for calibration, the audiologist first ascertains that the appropriate pressure microphone for earphone calibration is in place on the SPLM. The pistonphone, emitting a signal of calibrated frequency and intensity, is attached to the microphone of the SPLM and is used to make certain that SPLM readings in dB SPL are accurate. If readings are not accurate, the SPLM may undergo minor screwdriver adjustments prior to the calibration process such that pistonphone readings are accurate. Couplers are pieces of equipment designed to accurately measure transducer responses. In this example, the correct coupler type is an NBS 9-A (ANSI S3.7-1995 [R2003]), also called an artificial ear or 6-cc coupler because it simulates average volume between the earphone diaphragm and the tympanic membrane (Corliss & Burkhard, 1953). This piece of equipment is carefully attached to the SPLM. The standardized procedure dictates that controls of the audiometer emit a pure-tone signal at 70 dB HL in a "continuously on" presentation mode, with the intensity dial remaining at this level throughout the process. The audiologist detaches the appropriate earphone from its accompanying headband and places it on top of the 6-cc coupler that also contains a specialized microphone. A weight of 500 grams holds the earphone in proper place and exerts a standardized force that simulates that of the headband. The audiometer is then "coupled" to the SPLM and the audiologist prepares to take audiometer output measurements from the SPLM. As the audiometer is calibrated in dB HL and readings are made in dB SPL, the audiologist makes corrections using the appropriate Reference Equivalent Threshold Sound Pressure Level (RETSPL) correction values for the specific transducer. These correction values are added to the 70 dB HL output, to arrive at the anticipated measurement in dB SPL for each frequency. Figure 3–10 shows major pieces of calibration equipment, with a portable audiometer coupled to a SPLM via a 6-cc coupler.

The audiologist sweeps through the discrete audiometric frequencies to take readings from the SPLM, making certain that its octave band filter also reflects the appropriate frequency. Some SPLMs display a digital reading of dB SPL, whereas others display values on a volume unit (VU) meter that incorporates a broad dB scale

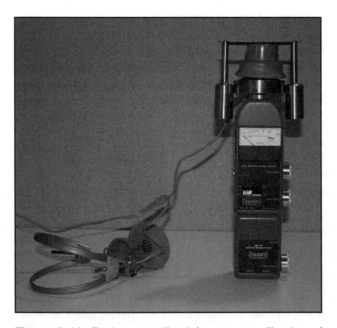

Figure 3–10. Equipment utilized for output calibration of audiometer.

in 10 dB steps and a finer dB scale in less than 1 dB steps. The audiologist's worksheet consists of "actual" intensity readings in dB SPL, as a function of frequency, and "ideal" intensity readings that represent an audiometer in perfect calibration. These "ideal" readings reflect the appropriate RETSPL reading for that specific transducer and frequency that is added to the base 70 dB HL audiometer dial reading. A comparison is made between the output that should be present versus the output that is actually measured.

The next step is to prepare a column of numbers that reflect differences between the actual and ideal values. It is beneficial to first determine if the actual audiometer intensity emitted is less than or greater than ideal values; that is, it is determined whether the audiometer's output is too intense or not intense enough. It is helpful to carry over the "+" or "−" sign prior to calculating the difference values. Once the difference values are calculated, the audiologist compares them to tolerance ranges specified by ANSI for that particular audiometer and frequency. If output is within the tolerance range at a particular frequency, the process is complete and no corrections must be made when recording results. If the difference is outside the tolerance range, however, the audiologist rounds the difference value to the nearest 5 dB and may construct a correction chart for use during pure-tone audiometry. The rounding occurs because pure-tone audiometry is performed in 5 dB steps. Table 3–1 shows a sample worksheet that illustrates this process and that the audiologist may utilize to determine if the audiometer is in proper calibration for output. This table is limited to the main audiometric frequencies for simplicity. The "Should Be" column provides the 70 dB HL constant plus the appropriate RETSPL value, to arrive at the anticipated dB SPL value. The "Actual" column provides the actual SPLM reading. Differences between "Should Be" and "Actual" values are shown. The "Within Tolerances" column implements ANSI's recommended plus or minus 3 dB allowance from 125 to 5 kHz and plus or minus 5 dB allowance at 6 kHz or higher. The final "Correction" column provides rounded values to be transferred to a correction chart.

Table 3–1. Example of Worksheet Utilized for Output Calibration of Audiometers

Frequency	TDH 49	Should Be	Actual	Difference	W/in Tolerance?	Correction
250 Hz	26.5	96.5	90.0	−6.5	No	−5 dB
500 Hz	13.5	83.5	86.0	+2.5	Yes	None
1 kHz	7.5	77.5	81.5	+4.0	No	+5 dB
2 kHz	11.0	81.0	79.5	−1.5	Yes	None
4 kHz	10.5	80.5	76.0	−4.5	No	−5 dB
8 kHz	13.0	83.0	79.0	−4.0	Yes	None

The clinician either adds or subtracts the designated correction value in dB at that particular frequency to the audiometer dial reading on obtaining and then recording threshold. Although appearing counterintuitive at first, the audiologist must add to the dial reading when the audiometer intensity is "too intense" and must subtract to the dial reading when the audiometer intensity is "not intense enough." For example, if a patient's true threshold is 30 dB HL and the audiometer is emitting 10 dB more intensity than it should, the following scenario would occur during testing, as illustrated in Table 3–2.

The patient would not respond at a 10 dB HL intensity dial reading (that is actually 20 dB HL) but would respond at a 20 dB HL dial reading (that is actually 30 dB HL). The tester would then need to add +10 dB to the dial reading to record the accurate threshold of 30 dB HL. One may proceed through a similar clinical scenario with an audiometer that is emitting intensity levels that are lower than expected and an example of this scenario is also illustrated in Table 3–2.

Table 3–2. Example of Threshold Determination When Audiometer Is Not in Proper Calibration According to Output

Audiometer emitting 10 dB "too much" True threshold = 30 dB HL		
Audiometer Dial Reading	*Actual Output*	*+ or – Patient Response*
0 dB HL	10 dB HL	–
10 dB HL	20 dB HL	–
20 dB HL	30 dB HL	+

The Audiologist must add +10 dB to the dial reading of 20 dB HL, in order to record threshold.

Audiometer emitting 10 dB "too little" True threshold = 30 dB HL		
Audiometer Dial Reading	*Actual Output*	*+ or – Patient Response*
10 dB HL	0 dB HL	–
20 dB HL	10 dB HL	–
30 dB HL	20 dB HL	–
40 dB HL	30 dB HL	+

The Audiologist must subtract 10 dB from the dial reading of 40 dB HL, in order to record threshold.

The audiologist repeats the calibration procedure for all other transducers: insert earphones, bone conduction vibrator, and loudspeaker system. The proper coupler to use with insert earphones is a 2-cc coupler, whereas the proper coupler to use with a bone conduction vibrator is an artificial mastoid. The audiologist utilizes the SPLM with a free-field microphone, instead of a pressure microphone, for measuring in the free field and must also utilize the appropriate transducer Reference Equivalent Threshold SPL corrections when converting from dB HL to dB SPL. Standards with regard to loudspeaker measurement specify azimuth, or relationship angle between listener and speaker, and whether listening is monaural or binaural.

The audiologist must also check calibration of the frequency parameter, through use of coupling the above described pieces of equipment to a digital frequency counter. The discrete frequencies noted on the audiometer's frequency dial are the "ideal" values, whereas the digital frequency readings are the "actual" values. The audiologist again utilizes ANSI procedures to determine if the actual measured value is within acceptable tolerances ranges. Tolerances vary according to audiometer type, but are generally within plus or minus 1 to 3% of the center audiometric frequency. For example, if a 3% criterion is used, a pure-tone signal intended to be 1 kHz may be measured within an acceptable range of 970 to 1030 Hz. One may note that the tolerance range varies from frequency to frequency, with a narrower tolerance range existing at lower frequencies and higher tolerance range existing at higher frequencies. If the frequency measurement is outside tolerance, a correction sheet may not be constructed for frequency because of the discrete, as opposed to continuous, nature of the frequency dial. The audiometer must be sent to the manufacturer or otherwise brought into compliance.

Although checking calibration for frequency and intensity are primary areas, the above descriptions represent only the "tip of the iceberg." The audiologist must check for attenuator linearity, to make certain that intensity is increasing in the desired increments. When a pure tone is emitted, the clinician must check to ensure that it is indeed a pure tone with no harmonics or harmonic distortion present. Harmonic frequencies are multiples of the fundamental frequency and, if present, the listener could potentially be responding to them. Signals and switches must be checked for various aspects, including rise and fall times of the signals, and presence of unwanted noise. Narrow band, speech, and white noise channels must be properly calibrated for intensity and frequency band represented, so that accurate usage in the clinic may be ensured. Calibration of non-traditional audiometers, such as automatic and speech audiometers, must also take place. Immittance audiometers must be calibrated on a regular basis, including the pure-tone signals that they emit, as must all other equipment housed within the audiology clinic. As previously discussed, the clinician must also make ambient noise measures within the sound suite to make certain that they are in compliance with maximum permissible levels. Although an extensive discussion of calibration procedures is beyond the scope of this textbook, one may easily see the importance of properly calibrating equipment and the challenges present in making accurate measurements. The reader is encouraged to refer to ANSI standards for detailed descriptions and the audiology student is encouraged to gain valuable hands-on experiences in this critical area.

THE DAILY LISTENING CHECK

In addition to yearly or otherwise regular calibration, the clinician should implement daily listening checks prior to testing patients. Many audiologists have developed their own protocols, often requiring a listener and a manipulator of controls. The audiologist should ensure that all cords are intact with no fraying. All equipment should be plugged in with jacks inserted into the proper jack panel section. A continuous tone may be presented to the listener at a comfortable listening level, while the frequency dial is manipulated to ensure proper changes in pitch. Similarly, linearity of the attenuator dial may be examined at various frequencies, to gauge increments in approximate 10 dB steps. All transducers should be checked for proper emission of the signal, cross-talk, and any extraneous noise. Table 3–3 illustrates a comprehensive daily listening check checklist.

Table 3–3. Major Areas to Include in Daily Listening Checks

• Making certain all jacks and pieces of equipment are properly plugged in

• Checking all transducer and other cords for fraying: this may be accomplished by moving the cords a section at a time while listening to a continuous tone

• Making certain that all transducers are in good working order: for example, that earphones are properly mounted in cushions and that insert earphones are properly coupled to cords. One should also check the bone conduction vibrator and the speaker system

• Listening via all transducers as one sweeps through the frequencies: the intensity may be a comfortably loud level and, although one is not expected to demonstrate perfect pitch, one should hear the pitch becoming higher. The tone should not sound intermittent and the audiologist(s) should also listen to FM and pulsed signals for accuracy.

• Making certain that no other noise is heard through the transducers when a signal is presented

• Making certain that a signal is presented to one ear only and that no cross-talk is present

• Frequency sweep described above should also be performed with narrow bands of noise and the listener should also listen to white noise/speech noise channels.

• Placing the frequency dial at 1 kHz and presenting signals of various intensities, raising in 10 dB steps: although one is not expected to exactly identify 10 dB steps, one should note the intensity becoming louder.

• Double checking the microphone of the audiometer for monitored live voice testing, the microphone located inside the booth to hear patient responses, and the talk back system so that the audiologist and patient may communicate.

• Checking the interruptor switch so that noise is not present when a signal is presented

• Checking the speech circuitry, CDs, and CD player for proper usage

• Making certain that there is no electrical interference, that ventilation is adequate, that the sound suite is comfortable for the patient, and that ambient noise is minimal

• Checking all other pieces of equipment to ensure proper function: otoscopes, immittance audiometer, hearing aid measurement equipment, electrophysiology equipment, equipment for vestibular evaluation, and others.

PATIENT PREPARATION

A patient may be referred as an inpatient or outpatient for a variety of complaints. Procedures described for patient preparation primarily pertain to the adult or older child population, with whom conventional techniques are used. Techniques for more challenging populations appear in a later section (see Chapter 7). Prior to pure-tone testing, the audiologist establishes rapport and elicits thorough case history information. Through the case history process, the audiologist gains important information regarding hearing and other ear-related complaints, medical history, previous ear surgery, communication history, employment, and recreational history. It is important for the interviewer to inquire about previous audiologic evaluations, hearing aid usage, surgeries, aural rehabilitation, and other relevant areas. It is also important to obtain previous records so that the patient's file may be thorough and so that current results may be compared with past results.

The audiologist also performs an otoscopic examination bilaterally. He or she learns techniques to help straighten the S-shaped ear canal, often by pulling upward and backward on the pinna, in a diagonal manner for optimum visualization of the external ear canal and tympanic membrane. The clinician should be well versed regarding major landmarks of the pinna and external auditory canal, so that any abnormalities may be identified. The audiologist also learns to identify collapsing ear canals by exerting slight pressure on the pinna prior to the otoscopic examination, to determine closure of the ear canal with such pressure. If this occurs, effects of collapsed canals may be alleviated through use of insert earphones. The beginning clinician should also be able to visualize the tympanic membrane and any occlusions, such as cerumen, that are present within the ear canal. If cerumen is occluding, the blockage should be removed prior to testing so that accurate test results may be obtained. If not properly removed prior to testing, inaccurate interpretations may be made regarding presence, severity and/or type of hearing impairment and inappropriate recommendations made.

The audiologist checks for a normal, pearly gray tympanic membrane color and for its typically visible landmarks, such as the cone of light and the manubrium of the malleus. As the clinician gains additional experience, he or she will become well versed in identifying such entities as ear canal lesions, foreign bodies, abnormal tympanic membrane color, bulging or retracted tympanic membrane, perforations, fluid within the middle ear space, and many others. Certain phenomena are red flags for referral to a physician and these include: blood located within the ear canal or behind the tympanic membrane, drainage, ear pain or otalgia, lesions or sores, sudden hearing loss, tinnitus, and dizziness.

In accompanying the patient into the sound suite, most audiologists arrange furniture so that the patient may not look directly at the window and the examiner. Patients facing the examiner may perceive subtle facial expressions or other cues that may designate when a tone has been presented and when he or she should respond. For proper transducer placement, earrings, hats, other head coverings, glasses, chewing gum and any other food items are removed. Hearing aids and other amplification systems are left intact during instructions, so that the patient may hear, and then are removed prior to transducer placement. If possible, earphone cords should be placed in back of the patient so that they do not interfere with testing by distracting or creating unnecessary noise. Because initial pure-tone tests involve listening to very soft sounds for obtaining thresholds, all other noises and modes of potential interference should be minimized and the patient should remain quiet. It is important to explain procedures step-by-step to each patient, in an individualized manner and so that instructions are well understood. Prior to pure-tone testing with an adult or older child who will be tested via conventional techniques, variations on the following instructions are provided:

> I am going to place these earphones (or inserts) on (or in) your ears. You will hear some tones (beeps) that will be very soft. Please press

this button each time you hear the sound, even if it is very soft. I will be testing your right (or better) ear first and will let you know when we will be switching to the other side. Do you have any questions?

Common responses may also be to ask the patient to raise a hand on hearing the tone, or even to indicate a positive response by saying "yes." The audiologist informs the patient that the door of the testing suite will be closed and that he or she will be seated at equipment on the other side of the window. To ensure patients' comfort levels, they are reassured that they and the examiner will be able to communicate throughout the testing session, although they should try to remain very quiet during this section of the testing session. It is important to remain in close communication with the patient, through use of the talk-back system, and to carefully instruct the patient during each step of the diagnostic process.

INFECTION CONTROL

Infection control in the audiology clinic is very important, in order to control the spread of disease from individual to individual or from work environment to individual. It is recommended that each clinic devise its own infection control plan and carefully implement these guidelines. Clinicians handle many items, such as earmolds and hearing aids, which may contain harmful bacteria and other organisms. Otoscope specula, earphones, immittance probe tips, cerumen removal curettes, and other items may be used with multiple patients and infection precautions must be taken. Diabetic, elderly, pediatric, HIV-positive, and other immunocompromised patients may especially be at risk if proper precautions are not taken in the clinic. One of the most basic procedures that an audiologist must implement is frequent hand-washing with antibacterial soap and water, immediately prior to and after each patient visit, as many diseases may be transmitted through direct contact.

The audiologist frequently encounters cerumen during the otoscopic examination and pure-tone testing, especially when insert earphones are utilized. The audiologist must exercise caution such that the insert does not further impact the cerumen and such that the earphone sound openings remain patent. According to Kemp et al. (1996), cerumen should be treated as an infectious agent because the clinician may not visually determine cerumen content and possible bodily fluid contamination in an accurate manner. Gloves should be worn when the clinician is exposed to cerumen and/or other bodily fluids. Safety glasses and masks may be in order if cerumen irrigation is taking place, as well as during the grinding and buffing process of hearing aids and earmolds, as splash-backs may occur. The audiologist should make certain that instruments containing cerumen or blood are disposed of in a careful manner.

Disinfecting agents kill germs and hospital-quality disinfectants should be used within the audiology clinic. Items that should be disinfected after cleaning include: specula, earphones, and hearing aid earmolds, as well as working area surfaces and pediatric setting toys. Sterilization involves killing all harmful microorganisms with each application and items such as specula, immittance probe tips, and cerumen removal instrumentation should be sterilized after cleaning (Kemp & Bankaitis, 2000). Infection control protocols and their importance within the audiology clinic cannot be overestimated, so that optimum hearing health care may be provided.

REFERENCES

American National Standards Institute. (2004). *Specifications for audiometers (S3.6-2004)*. New York: Acoustical Society of America.

Corliss, E. L. R., & Burkhard, M. D. (1953). A probe tube method for the transfer of threshold standard between audiometer earphones. *Journal of the Acoustical Society of America, 25*, 990–993.

Decker, T. N. (1990). *Instrumentation: an introduction for students in the speech and hearing sciences.* New York: Longman.

Frank, T., & Rosen, A. D. (2007). Basic instrumentation and calibration. In R. Roeser, M. Valente, & H. Hosford-Dunn (Eds.), *Audiology diagnosis* (2nd ed., pp. 195–237). New York: Thieme.

Kemp, R. J., & Bankaitis, A. E. (2000). Infection control for audiologists. In H. Hosford-Dunn, R. Roeser, & M. Valente (Eds.), *Audiology diagnosis, treatment and practice management* (Vol. III, pp. 257–279). New York: Thieme.

Kemp, R. J., Roeser, R. J., Pearson, D. W., & Ballachandra, B. B. (1996). *Infection control for the professions of audiology and speech language pathology.* Olathe, KS: Iles.

Killion, M. L. (1984). New insert earphones for audiometry. *Hearing Instruments, 35,* 38–46.

4 *Threshold*

Methods of Ascertaining and Recording

From a hearing science perspective, threshold is defined as the softest level of a specified signal that may be audible to the listener or that may evoke an auditory sensation. The ear is a nonlinear organ, such that it is not equally sensitive across frequencies. Specifically, less pressure is required in normal listeners to reach threshold from 1000 to 3000 Hz than at higher and lower frequencies. Threshold measurements in diagnostic audiology are the basis for air and bone conduction pure-tone audiometry. Audiologists' definitions of threshold may slightly vary from those used by psychoacousticians, in that audiologists typically measure patient response levels in 5 dB steps. The audiologist's clinical procedure may be streamlined in comparison to more precise protocols utilized in the laboratory, so that the clinical practice runs smoothly and is time efficient. Many factors may affect threshold, such as stimulus used, its duration, stimulus on and off times, time interval between stimuli, and presentation pattern. In addition to these variables that may affect threshold, results also may be affected by ambient noise levels, methodology, decibel increments, instructions provided, patient variables, examiner variables, and numerous other entities.

Although manipulation of equipment dials seems straightforward, it is the audiologist's responsibility to control for variability and obtain the most accurate possible results. These protocols are utilized to generate symbols recorded on an audiogram, which in turn are interpreted with regard to various parameters of hearing impairment. Threshold may be slightly variable in the same listener from one moment to the next (Green & Swets, 1974). In order to quantify this measurement and to develop standardized testing procedures, threshold from a clinical perspective is defined as the softest signal that a person may hear and therefore provide some type of response, at least 50% of the time. In basic hearing science and audiology courses, the student learns various methods that have historically been used to attain threshold with research subjects and clinical patients.

PSYCHOPHYSICAL METHODS

Method of Adjustment

The method of adjustment is a psychophysical method that is used primarily to determine thresholds (Yost, 2000). With this method, oftentimes used in automatic audiometry, the patient varies the stimulus to match a predetermined criterion. Instructions are for the patient to push a button when he or she hears the stimulus, at which time the signal intensity begins to attenuate. When the stimulus is no longer audible, the patient is asked to release the response button, at which time the signal becomes louder in intensity. This process is continued while the patient listens to continuous tones of either discrete or continuous frequency and the patient's threshold is bracketed. An example of automatic audiometry use is in industry, when the audiologist may wish to test numerous patients simultaneously.

A tracking or Békésy procedure is a variation of the method of adjustment, where the patient automatically presses a button as long as a tone is heard and releases the button when the signal is inaudible. In this manner, a tracing is made of threshold and threshold is ascertained as the mid- or 50% point of intensity excursion height as frequency is swept. The method of adjustment may also be utilized in other audiologic tasks, such as comparing two stimuli for perception of equal loudness or to discover a just noticeable difference with regard to frequency, intensity, or time. In these instances, stimulus No. 1 is a reference that remains constant while stimulus No. 2 is varied by the subject until the desired criterion is reached.

Method of Constant Stimuli

The method of constant stimuli is another psychophysical method used to obtain threshold (Yost, 2000). Continuously present stimuli range from rarely to always perceivable and many are presented, one at a time. The patient responds to each presentation, according to a predesignated criterion. For example, in ascertaining threshold, he/she may simply respond positively or negatively to indicate whether the stimulus was heard. This method of ascertaining threshold may be utilized in research, due to the large number of stimulus presentations and often smaller than 5 dB steps utilized. A precise threshold measure may be determined, using the criterion of "softest level at which the patient hears the stimulus 50% of the time." With regard to other tasks that compare two stimuli, such as loudness matching or finding just noticeable differences, the patient may provide responses indicating that one stimulus is "equal to" or "higher/lower than" another.

Method of Limits

The method of limits is a third psychophysical method for determining threshold and is used most often in diagnostic audiology. With this method, stimuli are introduced to the patient and controlled by the clinician. Stimulus parameters are varied by the examiner, based on patient response to previous stimuli presentation. For example, when the audiologist is obtaining threshold, a pure-tone is presented at a certain intensity level, based on the patient's previous response. If the patient responds positively to a stimulus, the subsequent signal presentation is lower in intensity; if the patient does not respond to a stimulus, the subsequent signal presentation is higher in intensity. In this manner, the audiologist may also bracket threshold. This method may also be utilized for additional types of tasks, such as judging two signals that are equal in loudness or that are just noticeably different with respect to a specific parameter. One may readily note that a subjective response is required, such as raising a hand or providing a verbal response, in order to obtain valid measures.

Modified Hughson-Westlake Procedure

Most audiologists utilize the modified Hughson-Westlake Procedure during pure-tone testing, first described by Hughson and Westlake (1944) and Carhart and Jerger (1959). These procedures first appeared in American National Standards Institute's published methods for manual pure-tone audiometry in 1978 (ANSI, 2004). Furthermore, the American Speech-Language-Hearing Association (ASHA) adapted guidelines devised by its Working Group on Manual Pure-Tone Threshold Audiometry in November, 1977. Updated Guidelines for Manual Pure-Tone Threshold Audiometry were approved by ASHA's Legislative Council in November, 2005.

Descending methods for obtaining threshold have been utilized, whereby the initial stimulus is audible to the patient and subsequent stimuli decrease in intensity. An advantage is that the patient is familiarized with the stimulus and "what to listen for," whereas a disadvantage is that false positive responses may result (patient response when no stimulus is presented). A subsequent section will address techniques the examiner may use to minimize false positive responses and obtain a valid/reliable audiogram, including varying presentation rate and rhythm. An ascending method, conversely, involves beginning stimulus presentation at a subaudible level and gradually increasing intensity in order to bracket threshold. One disadvantage of this technique may be difficulty conditioning the patient to the task required. Initial responses may be minimal response levels, as opposed to accurate thresholds. That is, the patient may wait to respond until the stimulus is "louder" or until "he is certain he hears it," as opposed to responding at the very softest audible level.

The following described Hughson-Westlake pure-tone threshold audiometric procedure is utilized in many clinics. It involves a combination of descending and ascending techniques to establish threshold. Specifically, the initial presentation is typically at a suprathreshold level. Intensity is decreased by 10 dB following a positive patient response and is increased by 5 dB following no response from the patient. The clinician seeks the softest level at which the patient responds at least 50% of the time. With some patients, especially those who may prove to be challenging cases, behavioral results may not represent true threshold or the softest sound heard. Rather, the clinician's judgment is that results represent minimal response levels (MRLs) that are indicative of the softest level at which a definitive response is observed.

THE AUDIOGRAM

Forms

A standard audiogram form is shown in Figure 4-1, although such forms may vary slightly from clinic to clinic. It incorporates recommendations first initiated by ANSI (1978) that the grid display "Frequency in Hertz (Hz)" logarithmically across the abscissa and "Hearing Level (HL) in Decibels (dB)" along the ordinate. The grid

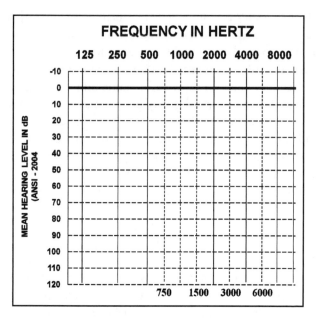

Figure 4–1. The audiogram form.

should be uniformly constructed according to a specific aspect ratio: the width designating one octave on the frequency scale should correspond in span to the length of 20 dB on the HL scale. Audiometric zero should be shown prominently across the frequency range, as compared to other intensity levels. Represented frequencies should be from at least 125 to 8000 Hz, whereas the dB levels should range from at least −10 dB to 120 dB HL. Some audiogram forms may display intensity levels higher than 120 dB HL, if the accompanying audiometer is capable of producing those levels.

An audiologist using ultrahigh-frequency audiometry may develop an audiogram form displaying these additional frequencies, keeping in mind the recommended logarithmic spatial representation of octave intervals.

Solid lines are utilized on the audiogram form to note octave frequency intervals, as well as 10 dB intensity increments. Dashed lines are utilized to note mid-octave frequencies of 750, 1500, 3000, and 6000 Hz. Clinics vary regarding identifying information included on the audiogram form, type of audiometer designation, patient reliability notation, and recording sections for other test results. Although some audiologists record right and left ear information on the same audiogram form, others choose to represent information from each ear on a separate audiogram as shown in Figure 4–2.

Some hearing clinics may also implement serial audiogram forms, which are useful with regular monitoring and numerous patient visits. These forms display frequency in Hz across the top, consistent with traditional forms. However, designators along the ordinate may simply note "R AC," "R BC," "L AC," and "L BC" to allow the audiologist to record numerical values of threshold in dB HL.

Audiometric Symbols

Audiometric symbols were constructed for simplicity and ease in discerning, for example, right ear from left ear responses, air conduction from bone conduction thresholds, and unmasked from masked thresholds. ASHA's Committee on Audiologic Evaluation presented guidelines for audiometric symbols in 1974 and a revised edition was adopted in 1989 (ASHA, 1990). Right ear thresholds are traditionally recorded in red, whereas left ear thresholds are recorded in blue. The audiologist may not rely on color differentiation or two-ear audiograms, as many clinics record two-ear information in the same color and on the same form. Air conduction (AC) symbols should be drawn on the audiogram so that the midpoint of the symbol is centered on the intersection of the appropriate frequency and intensity axes. The unmasked AC symbol for the right ear is an "O," whereas the symbol for the left ear is an "X." These symbols are reserved for situations when individual-ear information is obtained under earphones,

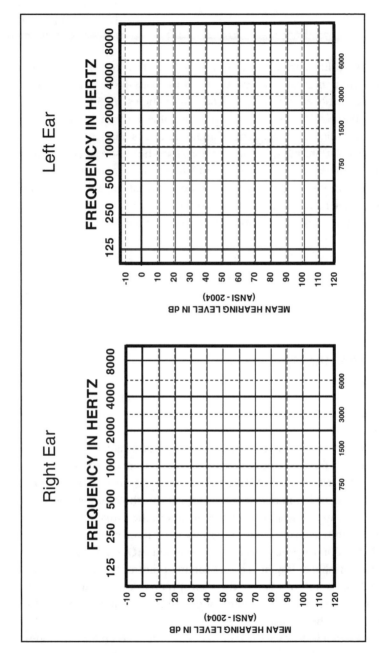

Figure 4–2. Two-ear audiogram form.

as opposed to within the sound field. Furthermore, these symbols represent the unmasked condition; that is, they were obtained in the test ear with no masking noise introduced to the nontest ear during testing. If the audiologist deems it necessary to place masking noise in the nontest ear while ascertaining AC threshold in the test ear, the following symbols are used: a red triangle for the right ear ($\triangle$) and a blue square for the left ear ($\square$). When clinical masking is performed during AC and/or BC testing, it is recommended that the audiologist also record the type and intensity levels of noise utilized to obtain thresholds and other results. All symbols should be recorded neatly and in uniform manner, with solid lines used to connect AC symbols of each ear. With recording of all symbols, the audiologist should keep in mind that the audiogram is a representation of himself or herself that is distributed to the professional community.

Disagreement has existed regarding representation of bone conduction (BC) thresholds. ASHA (1974) previously recommended using different symbols, depending on whether right or left mastoid process placement was used. Specifically, a red "<" was used to note the right ear threshold and a blue ">" was used to note the left ear threshold, when no masking noise was used in the nontest ear during testing. As previously discussed, pure-tones presented via BC stimulate both cochleas simultaneously; therefore, the above symbols represent transducer placement and not necessarily ipsilateral cochlear response. Alternative methods of recording BC thresholds have evolved and may be more highly recommended. Audiologists may plot unmasked BC thresholds in a manner denoting that the response is arising from an unspecified ear. Some audiologists may record unmasked thresholds using one of the already described BC symbols that denote transducer placement, whereas others may record such a response as an upside-down "V." When masking is used in the nontest ear, the right ear BC response is noted as a red, "[" whereas the masked BC response for the left ear is noted as a blue "]". BC symbols for the right ear should be placed on the left side of the frequency line at the appropriate intensity, with the open side close to but not touching the frequency line. Symbols for the left ear should be placed on the right side, with the open side close to but not touching the frequency line. If forehead placement is used, a "V" may denote an unmasked threshold, whereas a partial bracket such as ( ]) for the right and (⌈) for the left notes a masked threshold. BC symbols are typically not connected with a line, although some audiologists may connect them with a dashed line when significant air-bone gaps (ABG) are present. ABGs exist when AC thresholds are greater than 10 dB poorer than BC thresholds of the same ear and are determined frequency by frequency.

As with all symbols, uniformity and neatness should be preserved when recording on the audiogram. When unmasked or masked AC symbols are identical for the two ears, symbols may overlap. When the BC symbol is identical to the AC symbol, the former should be placed adjacent to but not touching the latter.

Occasionally, it becomes necessary to obtain thresholds within the sound field, such as with pediatric patients who do not accept earphones. Although no standardized symbol currently exists, many audiologists use an "S" to record these thresholds. These results must be carefully interpreted, since the testing session did not yield individual ear information and the recorded threshold may reflect performance of a better ear.

The audiologist may reach the intensity limit of the equipment while testing, via either AC or BC. When this occurs, the appropriate symbol is recorded and an arrow is attached at the bottom. For example, O, X, [, and] with attached arrows represent that limits were reached with no response via unmasked right AC, unmasked left AC, masked right BC, and masked left BC, respectively.

Various clinics may also develop other forms of nonstandardized audiogram symbols for their own personal use. It may be common to see "L" or "R" recorded on an audiogram to show left or right hearing aid responses within the sound field, or to see "CI" to note benefit received from a cochlear implant. Jerger (1976) described

Table 4–1A. Key of Major Audiometric Symbols

Audiogram Key		
	Right Ear	*Left Ear*
AC Unmasked	0	X
AC Masked	△	□
BC Unmasked (mastoid)	<	>
BC Masked (mastoid)	[	]
BC Unmasked (forehead)	V	
BC Masked (forehead)	]	[
Sound Field	S	

Table 4–1B. Key of Major Audiometric Symbols: Beyond the Equipment Limits

Audiogram Key		
	Right Ear	*Left Ear*
AC Unmasked	0↙	X↘
AC Masked	△↙	□↘
BC Unmasked (mastoid)	<↙	>↘
BC Masked (mastoid)	]↙	]↘
BC Unmasked (forehead)	V↓	
BC Masked (forehead)	]↙	[↘
Sound Field	S↓	

additional options for reporting audiometric data in scholarly publications. Tables 4–1A and 4–1B demonstrate typical audiometric symbols that may appear within an audiogram key on clinical testing forms.

MANUAL PURE-TONE THRESHOLD AUDIOMETRIC PROCEDURES

ASHA Guidelines for Manual Pure-Tone Threshold Audiometry were devised by a special Working Group and approved in 2005, as a revision of guidelines adopted in 1977. Manual or conventional audiometry is described, as differentiated from automatic or computerized audiometry. Guidelines were established to include procedures for both AC and BC testing, in an attempt to standardize these protocols. In addition to describing preferred audiometric equipment, calibration, transducers, and test environment, the guidelines convey specific infection control recommendations. Suggested patient preparation procedures, including instructions, have been discussed in a previous section.

Air Conduction Testing

Air conduction testing is routinely performed as the first part of a comprehensive audiologic evaluation, most often using supra-aural or insert earphones. The audiologist should request that the patient remove food, chewing gum, earrings, glasses, and head coverings. The audiologist adjusts the earphone headband to its maximum length, places the earphones on each ear, and then adjusts the headband length to the patient's head size. The red earphone should cover the right ear and the blue earphone should cover the left, with the transducer diaphragms covering each ear canal opening. Cords are often placed in the back, when possible, so that they don't distract the patient or interfere with perception of soft sounds. An insert should be the correct size for the patient's ear canal and should be inserted into the ear canal with sufficient depth, allowing the foam plugs to expand for at least 30 seconds prior to testing.

The audiologist typically begins testing at 1 kHz, as the ear is quite sensitive at this particular frequency. The better ear is tested first, in the event that masking must be performed while testing the poorer ear; if ears are thought to be symmetric, the right ear is often tested first. ASHA (2005) recommends starting out with an ascending technique, although many audiologists present the first tone(s) at a suprathreshold level. Pure-tone stimuli should be of 1 to 2 seconds' duration and presentation pattern should be varied. Tones should be continuous, although some patients are more attentive with pulsed tones (Burk & Wiley, 2004). The modified Hughson-Westlake procedure involves a dual-part process: the clinician decreases the intensity of the tone by 10 dB when the patient responds positively and increases the intensity of the tone by 5 dB when the patient does not respond. The examiner continues to elicit patient responses in this manner until threshold is obtained, defined as the lowest dB level at which responses occur in at least 50% of a series of ascending trials. The minimum number of responses needed to record threshold is two positive out of three total responses. Table 4–2 demonstrates an example of the Hughson-Westlake procedure for ascertaining pure-tone threshold.

The audiologist records the right ear (or better ear) AC symbol of the attained threshold in dB HL on the audiogram form. This procedure is repeated for 2 kHz, 4 kHz, 8 kHz, 500 Hz, and 250 Hz. Some clinicians reestablish threshold at 1 kHz following obtaining of threshold at 8 kHz, because threshold at 1 kHz was the first one obtained. Re-establishing the threshold at 1 kHz helps the audiologist verify the reliability of patient responses. Some protocols may include testing mid-octave frequencies and/or obtaining threshold at 125 Hz.

Table 4–2. Demonstration of the Hughson-Westlake Procedure for Attaining Threshold				
Stimuli Presentation and Patient Responses				
50 dB HL	+			
45 dB HL				
40 dB HL		+		
35 dB HL			+	
30 dB HL		−	+	+	+
25 dB HL			−	−	−
20 dB HL				−	−

The audiologist then obtains AC thresholds for the left ear (or poorer ear) in the same manner: 1 kHz, 2 kHz, 4 kHz, 8 kHz, 500 Hz, and 250 Hz. The clinician may once again choose to retest at 1 kHz as a reliability measure. All results are also plotted on the audiogram form and determination is made regarding testing of mid-octave frequencies. Audiologists may vary the order of frequencies tested with no effect on test results; following specific frequency and ear order protocols is recommended, for standardization purposes and to minimize the risk of inadvertently omitting an important test component. Masking may be warranted during AC testing in some cases and is addressed in Chapter 6.

Testing Mid-Octave Frequencies

The audiologist may perform testing at 125 Hz, especially if a low-frequency hearing loss is present. Testing of mid-octave frequencies may be included in certain monitoring programs, such as with ototoxicity, other forms of medical management and hearing conservation.

Ascertaining of mid-octave thresholds helps to "fill in audiometric gaps" and better observe a more complete audiometric configuration. These additional data points provide the audiologist with more information related to the patient's hearing loss. When a 20 dB or more difference in threshold exists between two consecutive octave frequencies, the mid-octave frequency should be tested. The examiner may apply this rule and return to test these frequencies once the audiogram is constructed or he/she may see the need to test mid-octaves and do so as the testing session progresses. No mid-octave frequency exists between 250 and 500 Hz.

The Pure-Tone Average

Once AC testing is performed for both the right and left ears, and masking implemented when deemed necessary, the audiologist calculates a pure-tone average (PTA) for each ear. These calculations are made with AC thresholds. The standardized method for calculating a PTA is to take an average of three thresholds: dB HL levels at 500 Hz, 1 kHz, and 2 kHz. These frequencies have been selected as they have traditionally been termed "speech frequencies," even though some primarily consonant speech sounds are made up of higher frequency information. The following provides a calculation example for one ear:

$$\frac{[45 \text{ dB HL } (500 \text{ Hz}) + 50 \text{ dB HL } (1 \text{ kHz}) + 60 \text{ dB HL } (2 \text{ kHz})]}{3} =$$

$$155/3 = 52 \text{ dB HL}$$

The PTA is rounded to the nearest whole number: if the number following the decimal is a "6," then the clinician rounds upward and if the number is a "3," the clinician rounds downward. The purpose of the PTA is to help the audiologist determine severity of the hearing loss, if present, and to serve as a system of checks and balances throughout the comprehensive evaluation. This measure should correlate well (within 10 dB) with the Speech Recognition Threshold (SRT) for that ear.

On occasion, it becomes necessary to calculate a two-frequency pure-tone average (PTA). This is calculated when there is a 20 dB or more difference between two consecutive speech frequencies (500 Hz and 1 kHz and/or 1 kHz and 2 kHz). A clue as to when to take a two-frequency average lies in whether a mid-octave frequency of 750 Hz and/or 1500 Hz was tested, although these frequencies do not enter into calculations. When calculating a two-frequency PTA, the two better frequencies are averaged, even if they are not consecutive. This value should correlate well with the magnitude estimate of hearing loss and also with the SRT. An example of calculating a two-frequency PTA appears below. A two-frequency PTA is indicated because the difference in thresholds between 1 kHz and 2 kHz is 20 dB or greater. In this case, the audiologist would disregard the 70 dB threshold and average the other two threshold values:

$$30 \text{ dB HL (500 Hz)} + 45 \text{ dB HL (1 kHz)} + 70 \text{ dB HL (2 kHz)}$$

$$\frac{[(30 \text{ dB HL} + 45 \text{ dB HL})}{2} = 37.5 \text{ dB HL}$$

(rounded to 37 dB HL or 38 dB HL)

Bone Conduction Testing

Bone conduction is another avenue by which we hear sounds, where vibratory energy produces compressions in the skull bones and disturbances in the ossicular chain and inner ear. According to Zemlin (1998), bone conducted stimuli stimulate the basilar membrane of the inner ear in three ways: skull displacement, inertial lag of the ossicular chain, and the occlusion effect (OE). The OE is defined as an increase in intensity of a bone conducted stimulus perceived by the listener, caused by occlusion of the external ear canal.

BC testing is an integral component of the comprehensive, diagnostic evaluation and may be performed after AC testing or following speech audiometry. Often, the audiologist performs speech audiometry following AC testing as the necessary transducers are already in place.

The audiologist typically places the BC vibrator on the mastoid process in preparation for testing, although alternative placements have been utilized. The better ear is selected first if the audiologist plans to perform testing with placement on both mastoids, anticipating the performance of masking when testing the poorer ear. Some audiologists may perform BC testing with transducer placement on the poorer ear only, while preparing the patient for the masking process and for noise to be introduced to the better ear. With transducer placement, the audiologist makes certain that hair is not interfering and that the vibrator is not touching the pinna. It is helpful to place the flat portion of the vibrator on the mastoid bone first and then to secure the headband in a diagonal fashion. Instructions for obtaining threshold are the same as those utilized for AC testing. The audiologist instructs the patient that "this oscillator" will be placed behind the ear to deliver tones and that he or she should continue to respond, even if the stimuli are very soft. The patient should also respond positively, regardless of ear perceived as hearing the tone. The testing session begins with finding threshold at 1 kHz, followed by 2 kHz, 4 kHz, 500 Hz, and 250 Hz. As with AC testing, the audiologist may wish to re-establish threshold at 1 kHz to verify reliability of results. Note that BC testing is typically not performed above 4 kHz, due to transducer limitations at higher frequencies. Unmasked BC thresholds are recorded on the audiogram, in cases of ear symmetry and when superimposed with AC thresholds such that masking is not warranted. These symbols represent the ear of transducer placement. BC results are obtained for both ears and are marked accordingly on the audiogram forms, in cases where masking is necessary. The reader is referred to audiogram symbols shown in Tables 4–1A and 4–1B.

BC symbols are not usually connected with lines, although some audiologists connect with dashed lines when AC results are significantly poorer than BC results. Pure-tone averages are not calculated through use of BC thresholds, nor do BC thresholds assist in determination of hearing loss magnitude. The audiologist views AC and BC thresholds, as well as their relationships, in determining whether the hearing loss is symmetric. Comparison of AC with BC results is crucial as the audiologist makes interpretation regarding type of hearing loss: conductive, sensorineural, or mixed. With AC testing, one may recall that the stimulus is delivered through the outer, middle, and inner ear prior to ascending the central auditory nervous system. BC testing bypasses a part of that entire system (outer and middle ear) by delivering the signal directly to the cochlea of the inner ear and actually to both simultaneously. This determination of type of loss, in turn, carries significant clinical implications regarding course of treatment that is recommended for the patient.

Although mastoid placement of the BC vibrator seems to be the most common for pure-tone testing, challenges do exist with regard to correct placement on the mastoid process and maintaining placement during testing. Some audiologists utilize forehead placement with masking noise presented to the nontest ear. Although placement of the vibrator on the forehead is straightforward, there may be output limitations of the transducer and possible calibration challenges that arise. This is because traditional BC calibration involves measuring force levels through usage of an artificial mastoid coupler, in addition to a traditional SPLM. The Sensorineural Acuity Level (SAL) test is another measure often affiliated with bone conduction testing, in that it may provide diagnostic information regarding type of hearing loss, particularly when true BC thresholds are questioned. This measure and the masking procedure are discussed in Chapter 6.

OBTAINING A VALID AUDIOGRAM

The beginning clinician initially focuses on familiarization with equipment and the procedures for obtaining pure-tone thresholds. As those procedures become more automatic, including recording of results, the clinician then begins to fine-tune clinical insights related to interpretation. Although the audiology profession has developed standardized procedures, variability and artifact may be introduced into the testing session. Especially as many pure-tone threshold procedures are subjective, the audiologist must exert great effort to ensure validity and reliability of his or her measures. Validity relates to ensuring that the clinician is measuring what he intends to measure, whereas reliability relates to reducing error so that results are consistent from test session to test session. Artifact may be introduced into the test session by way of clinician, patient, stimulus, and environmental variables.

Clinician Variables

The clinician should be well educated with regard to audiologic procedures, including integration of rigorous course work and varied clinical practicum experiences. Practicum experience should include extensive work across audiology's scope of practice and with patients across the life span. With experience, the audiologist gains clinical insights that extend far beyond actual threshold-obtaining procedures and recording of symbols. For example, the audiologist may make educated guesses as to the type of hearing loss from case history information or as to audiometric configuration after obtaining only several thresholds. The audiologist enters each individualized test session with flexibility, ready to adapt techniques as deemed necessary for each particular patient. Using pure-tone audiometry as a base, the audiologist makes predictions regarding subsequent test results and recommendations. Although predictions may be inaccurate as cases are often not "textbook" ones, flexibility and adaptation to each individual patient may help to reduce error. Techniques that are successful with one patient may not be so with another. An easy rapport with patients helps the audiologist's testing session run smoothly.

The audiologist learns excellent time management skills in efficiently progressing through case history information and the testing session without forfeiting test result accuracy. Variability may be introduced into the testing session if the patient load is too great and the audiologist is too rushed. It is also crucial to gain all the relevant case history information from all members of the hearing health care team, including patient and family, prior to testing and making recommendations.

In addition to test protocol expertise, the audiologist must bear in mind that instructions may affect test results. Specifically with regard to pure-tone testing, different results may be obtained if the patient is instructed to "raise a hand when he hears the tone," as opposed to "raise a hand even if the tone is very soft." The audiologist monitors responses to make certain that they are time-locked, as opposed to too delayed or too rapid following tonal presentation. He or she utilizes the talk-back system to reinforce the patient and to provide instructions with each step. The audiologist also closely monitors patient well-being and attentiveness throughout the testing session. Finally, the audiologist is well versed with regard to utilizing masking procedures, so that accurate thresholds are obtained and the audiogram accurately interpreted.

Patient Variables

Testing techniques described thus far have been of a conventional nature, usually used with adult and older pediatric populations. The audiologist may encounter individuals who are unable to respond via hand-raising, button-pushing, or other conventional techniques. On the younger end of the age spectrum, it may become necessary to utilize pediatric techniques, such as Visual Reinforcement Audiometry (VRA) or Conditioned Play Audiometry (CPA). The former involves conditioning the child to lateralize toward a lighted toy on hearing a stimulus and the latter involves conditioning the child to perform a play activity (dropping a block into a box, for example), on hearing a stimulus. Patients, including those on the geriatric end of the age spectrum, may demonstrate cognitive deficits or slowed reaction times. These patients may require slower paces during the testing session, frequent breaks, and regular reinstruction.

The audiologist may encounter a variety of patient responses, some of which may require reinstruction. Just as the tones presented are brief, the patient response should be brief. The patient may require reinstruction if keeping a hand up or holding the button longer than necessary when responding. When responses are too delayed, the audiologist may ask the patient to respond as soon as he or she hears the stimulus. Many clinicians encounter patients who elect to talk during the testing session or even to provide ongoing narrative of what is heard, when, and how intense. In these cases, the audiologist should diplomatically remind the patient that tones are very soft and that talking could lead to missing one. Patient response should be overt enough so that the clinician may distinctly observe from the audiometer controls; for example, if a patient subtly raises a finger upon hearing the stimulus, it may be necessary for the audiologist to ask the patient to raise an entire hand. Finally, the audiologist is situated so that he or she may see the patient, facial expressions, and other responses. This is important so that behavioral responses to stimuli, other than the one requested, may be observed. Also, the audiologist may note factors that could interfere with the testing session, such as patient sleepiness, fatigue, inattentiveness, or illness.

Family members are often present during the testing session. If they become distracting for the patient, the audiologist may tactfully ask them to remain quiet or out of patient view. Disorders and patient illness may also affect the reliability of test results. For example, audiologists working within an inpatient facility may see patients who are undergoing chemotherapy, who have suffered from cerebrovascular accidents, who have head trauma, or who demonstrate a variety of other disorders. These patients may arrive at the clinic in wheelchairs, may be scheduling an audiology appointment around other appointments, and may not feel well. As audiologists also diagnose and treat many patients with vestibular disorders, one must bear in mind that patients may be experiencing dizziness and other symptoms during the testing session. Patient responses may be inconsistent during the testing session, from a variety of factors including tinnitus. When inconsistent and false positive responses occur, the clinician should reinstruct, present a louder-than-threshold stimulus to refamiliarize the patient with the task, and perhaps retest utilizing a frequency-modulated or pulsed tonal stimulus.

Stimulus Variables

The stimulus of choice for pure-tone testing is a continuous one, although the reader has seen that adaptations may be necessary and alternate forms of stimuli needed. When testing in the sound field, FM and/or pulsed tones are recommended for alleviation of standing waves. Such varied stimuli may also be more "interesting" for the pediatric patient than continuous tones. The recommended presentation length is 1 to 2 seconds, with longer or shorter durations potentially affecting test results. Results obtained during pure-tone testing should correlate well with those obtained during speech audiometry and other components of the testing session.

Proper calibration of equipment is essential, so that frequency and intensity of stimuli are as intended and as demonstrated on audiometer controls. The daily listening check is also important, to ensure equipment is functioning well and to eliminate effects of any earphone crosstalk or abnormal acoustic radiation from transducers. As the ear demonstrates greatest sensitivity at 1 kHz, this is often the first frequency tested. Threshold is re-established here and for any other frequency that may be deemed questionable after the initial trial. Masking noise circuitry should also be in proper calibration with proper procedures utilized, so that accurate thresholds are obtained in the test ear.

Environment Variables

The testing environment should be comfortable and accessible for the patient, so that he or she may concentrate on tasks required during the testing session. The sound suite should exude a professional appearance and should be free of auditory and visual distractions. Presence of extra equipment and supplies within the sound suite may affect calibration. The environment within the suite should adhere to maximum permissible noise levels as required by ANSI (2004). Environmental noise levels determine whether a single- or double-walled booth is necessary and the installers must also be aware of electrical interferences. Family members may be present for patient reassurance during testing, although they should remain quiet and out of the way. They should not provide clues to the patient or otherwise participate in the testing session. Similarly, the environment should be staged so that the patient does not derive clues from the examiner.

The sound suite should be large enough to accommodate its particular testing session. For example, the smallest booth available may accommodate conventional techniques whereas a larger suite is required for sound field work. Proper calibration should include stimuli presented via loudspeakers and the patient should be seated at the properly calibrated location when sound field testing is performed. The environment may be adapted for individual patient needs throughout the testing session. Although examples are endless, one example is to seat the claustrophobic patient so that he may see the examiner through the window or so that the door may be opened periodically throughout the testing session.

REFERENCES

American National Standards Institute. (1978). *Methods for manual pure-tone threshold audiometry* (ANSI S3.21-1978, R-1986). New York: Author.

American National Standards Institute. (2004). *Methods for manual pure-tone threshold audiometry* (ANSI S3.21-2004). New York: Author.

American Speech-Language-Hearing Association. (1974). Guidelines for audiometric symbols. *Asha, 16*, 260–264.

American Speech-Language-Hearing Association. (1990). *Guidelines for audiometric symbols*. Rockville, MD: Author.

American Speech-Language-Hearing Association. (2005). *Guidelines for manual pure-tone threshold audiometry*. Rockville, MD: Author.

Burk, M. H., & Wiley, T. L. (2004). Continuous versus pulsed tones in audiometry. *American Journal of Audiology, 13*, 54–61.

Carhart, R., & Jerger, J. (1959). Preferred method for clinical determination of pure-tone thresholds. *Journal of Speech and Hearing Disorders, 16*, 340–345.

Green, D. M., & Swets, J. A. (1974). *Signal detection theory and psychophysics*. New York: Wiley & Sons.

Hughson, W., & Westlake, H. D. (1944). Manual for program outline for rehabilitation of aural casualties both military and civilian. *Transactions of the American Academy of Ophthalmology and Otolaryngology, 48*(Suppl.), 1–15.

Jerger, J. (1976). Proposed audiometric symbol system for scholarly publications. *Archives of Otolaryngology, 102*, 33–36.

Yost, W. A. (2000). *Fundamentals of hearing: An introduction* (4th ed.). San Diego, CA: Academic Press.

Zemlin, W. R. (1998). *Speech and hearing science: Anatomy and physiology* (4th ed.). Boston: Bacon.

5 *Audiogram Interpretation*

Once the audiologist has obtained and recorded thresholds for each ear across the designated frequency range, he or she is faced with the important task of interpretation. As with any audiologic measure, mastering the testing procedure is only one of several important components. It is critical that audiologists master all procedures from straightforward to complex and even more important for him or her to make accurate interpretations resulting in quality hearing health care for the patient. Once AC and BC thresholds are recorded, the audiologist interprets the audiogram based on four major parameters: magnitude, type, configuration, and symmetry.

Magnitude

The first question the audiologist may ask is whether a hearing loss is present. If a hearing loss is present, it may appear in one or both ears. Most audiogram forms note a solid line at the lower limit of the normal hearing range, such that thresholds appearing at that level or better are considered to be within normal limits. Hearing loss severity is classified according to categories or ranges. If adults demonstrate hearing sensitivity within normal to borderline normal limits, this typically means that all AC thresholds are 20 to 25 dB HL or better at all test frequencies. Different criteria may be used with children, in that thresholds poorer than 15 dB HL may have significant impact on speech, language and academic development (Dobie & Berlin, 1979; Skinner, 1978). Adults may be considered by some audiologists to demonstrate a slight hearing impairment if thresholds appear between 16 to 25 dB HL. Other categories of hearing loss magnitude are as follows:

26 dB HL to 40 dB HL	Mild
41 dB HL to 55 dB HL	Moderate
56 dB HL to 70 dB HL	Moderately severe
71 dB HL to 90 dB HL	Severe
91+ dB HL	Profound

As a guideline in interpretation, it is important to determine magnitude by viewing AC thresholds and to consider the entire frequency range. For example, if one only views PTAs and interprets a hearing loss as "mild" (for example, with a PTA of 32 dB HL), this is not entirely accurate if the configuration sharply falls to the severe range in higher frequencies. Although practice is required for the student of Audiology, he or she should be as descriptive as possible during counseling and report writing explanations. The reader should be able to visualize the audiogram from verbal description or report wording, prior to actually viewing the audiogram form.

As one views serial audiograms of the same patient, one should look for diminished hearing as a function of frequency. As threshold is often 5 dB variable from one moment to the next, the clinician compares thresholds and views a 10 dB shift or greater as significant.

Type

Type of hearing loss is often one of the most difficult of interpretation parameters. The first type is a conductive hearing loss, where a disorder occurs within the outer and/or middle ear, impeding conduction of the stimulus through this part of the auditory system. Examples of the many common conductive disorders are otitis media, otosclerosis, ossicular chain disarticulation, and tympanic membrane perforation. As a general rule, a primary referral will be a medical one because these disorders are often medically or surgically treatable. The second type of hearing loss is a sensorineural hearing loss, where a disorder occurs within the inner ear or more central aspect of the auditory system. The "sensory" component of the term indicates a peripheral disorder often targeting hair cell function within the cochlea whereas the "neural" component indicates VIIIth nerve or other central pathology. Although beyond the scope of this textbook, the audiologist is well versed in various forms of differential diagnosis to help rule out central pathology. Examples of common cochlear disorders are presbycusis, Ménière's disease, noise-induced hearing loss, and hearing loss from ototoxic medications. An acoustic neuroma or VIIIth nerve tumor is an example of a more central or retrocochlear pathology. Although medical referrals are certainly in order with sensorineural losses, these hearing losses are typically not medically or surgically treatable and aural (re)habilitative strategies are recommended. For example, these patients may be prime candidates for hearing aids, cochlear implants, other hearing assistive technology, communication strategy training, and additional forms of rehabilitation. The third and final type of hearing loss discussed here is a mixed loss, where a disorder occurs in the conductive mechanism (outer and/or middle ear) and within the inner ear or central auditory system. An example lies in a patient who has presbycusis, sensorineural hearing loss as a result of aging, and who also demonstrates a conductive component caused by a tympanic membrane perforation. The primary referral is medical, for treatment of the conductive component, and then rehabilitative strategies are recommended to treat the residual sensorineural component. Many combinations of conductive and sensorineural pathologies may lead to display of a mixed hearing loss on the audiogram.

In order to determine type of hearing loss, the audiologist views AC and BC relationships recorded on the audiogram for the same ear, frequency by frequency. The following chart may assist in differentiating among the three major types of hearing impairment:

	Loss by AC?	Loss by BC?	Significant Air-Bone Gaps?
Conductive	yes	no	yes
Sensorineural	yes	yes	no
Mixed	yes	yes	yes

With regard to conductive loss, one may select an example disorder such as otitis media. As one builds on knowledge related to ear anatomy and air conduction testing, one may see that the pure-tone signal must be delivered through the entire peripheral system, including the middle ear where this disorder occurs. Therefore, a logical assumption is that there will be a hearing loss by air conduction (AC), visualized on the audiogram. When testing by bone conduction (BC), however, the examiner bypasses this middle ear disorder and delivers signals to the intact cochlea. Theoretically the patient should not exhibit a hearing loss by BC in this case. There will be significant air-bone gaps (ABGs), defined as >10 dB difference between AC and BC thresholds at any one frequency of the same ear. A significant ABG may also be defined as a 15 dB or greater difference between AC and BC thresholds as testing is accomplished in 5 dB steps. AC thresholds will be poorer than BC thresholds with a conductive hearing loss. In fact, AC should be poorer than or equal to

BC thresholds in any testing situation as the former evaluates the entire mechanism and the latter evaluates only a part of that mechanism. Very small bone-air gaps may occur (5-10 dB), where BC thresholds are poorer than AC thresholds, due to equipment/tester artifact or skull thickness but these results should be repeated; if such gaps are larger, additional troubleshooting is in order. The audiogram in Figure 5-1 demonstrates a conductive hearing loss in each ear. BC thresholds are masked, in the presence of significant ABGs.

With a sensorineural loss, such as that resulting from ototoxicity, one may also envision a hearing loss by AC as the signal is delivered through the entire peripheral mechanism that includes the inner ear. In once again visualizing ear anatomy and the BC testing process, one may reason that a hearing loss by BC should also be noted, as the signal is delivered directly to the cochlea where the disorder is present. In fact, AC and BC thresholds in this case should be superimposed and there should be no significant air bone gaps. Occasionally, one may see air bone gaps of 5 dB or 10 dB in these cases but these are not considered to be significant. These slight variations may occur because threshold is variable from one testing session/experience to the next and there are many extraneous factors that may affect threshold measurements. The audiogram in Figure 5-2 demonstrates a sensorineural hearing loss in each ear.

With a mixed hearing loss, such as may be seen with otitis media and presbycusis, one may readily see that a hearing loss will be apparent on the audiogram via AC testing. The AC signal will first be delivered through the middle ear, where the first disorder lies, and will then be delivered to the second disorder found in the cochlea. Signals delivered by BC testing will bypass the conductive mechanism and otitis media, but will be delivered to the presbycusic inner ear. Therefore, a hearing loss will also be demonstrated via BC thresholds. BC thresholds will be significantly better than those obtained by AC and significant ABGs will be seen on the audiogram. The audiogram in Figure 5-3 demonstrates a mixed hearing loss in each ear. BC thresholds are masked, in the presence of significant ABGs.

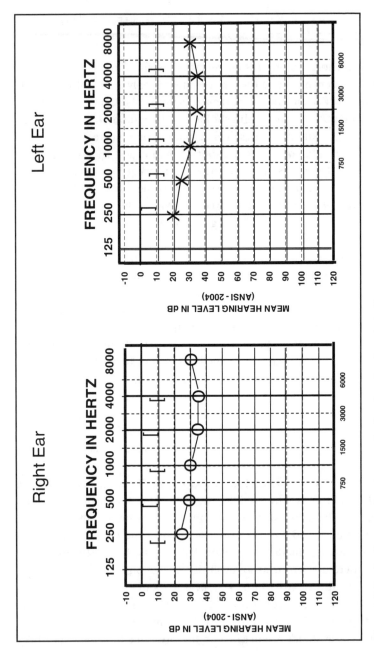

Figure 5–1. Audiogram showing conductive hearing loss in both ears.

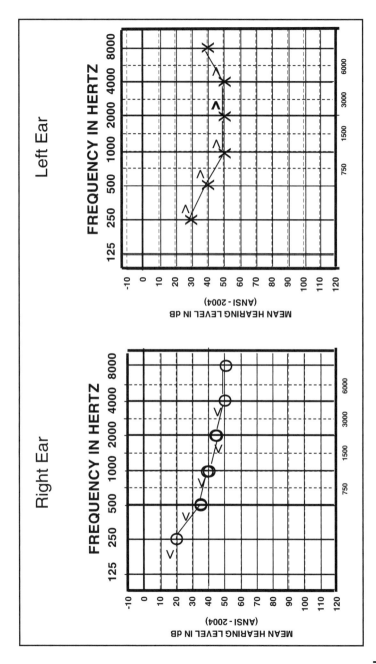

Figure 5–2. Audiogram showing sensorineural hearing loss in both ears.

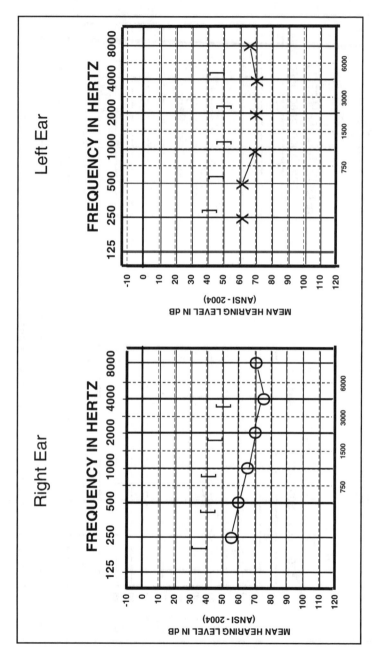

Figure 5–3. Audiogram showing mixed hearing loss in both ears.

In comparing conductive and mixed hearing losses, both demonstrate ABGs, but BC thresholds are within normal limits with conductive losses. With regard to sensorineural and mixed losses, both demonstrate losses by both AC and BC, but there are significant ABGs with a mixed loss. Audiograms may show an endless variety of results. There may be a hearing loss of one type in one ear and of another type in the other ear. There may be ABGs at some frequencies and not at others. Hearing loss may not be the same magnitude at all frequencies and masking may be required at only some frequencies.

Configuration

The third interpretation parameter discussed here is configuration or audiometric shape, assessed by viewing AC thresholds of each ear. Although configurations are not quantified to the degree that other audiologic measures are, below are general terms and guidelines (Stach, 1998):

Flat	Thresholds are within 20 dB of each other across frequency range
Rising	Thresholds at low frequencies are at least 20 dB poorer than at high frequencies
Sloping	Thresholds at high frequencies are at least 20 dB poorer than at low frequencies
Precipitous	Thresholds are steeply sloping (at least 20 dB/octave) in higher frequencies

Low-frequency losses may exist that are limited to the low-frequency region or high-frequency losses may exist that are limited to that portion of the frequency range. The audiologist may also see trough-shaped configurations where thresholds at 1000 and 2000 Hz are significantly poorer than those in lower and higher frequencies. An inverted trough-shaped configuration indicates that sensitivity at these middle frequencies is significantly better than sensitivity in lower and higher frequencies. Finally, a configuration may not fit these patterns and may be considered S-shaped, jagged in configuration, or verbally described on a frequency-by-frequency basis.

Configuration is an important aspect of the hearing loss to consider, in that this parameter provides clues regarding hearing disorder. For example, the audiologist may suspect presbycusis with a bilateral sensorineural hearing loss that is symmetric and gradually falling in configuration. A unilateral, rising sensorineural hearing loss may be an indication of Ménière's disease whereas a bilateral sensorineural hearing loss that notches in configuration at 4 kHz may be an indication of noise exposure. Through extensive education and experience, the audiologist integrates configuration and other important diagnostic information to gain clues regarding hearing loss etiology.

Knowledge of hearing loss configuration also provides crucial information toward the audiologic rehabilitation process. After viewing audiogram characteristics including configuration, the audiologist makes educated guesses regarding expected word recognition abilities. Speech understanding abilities are affected by audiometric configuration, with one example being the patient with a high-frequency sensorineural hearing loss who experiences difficulty discriminating high-frequency phonemes. As the audiologist superimposes the audiogram on a diagram of the average speech spectrum, he or she may determine how well the patient is receiving average conversational speech and how well the patient is discriminating various speech sounds.

Audiogram configuration also is a major consideration in selection of amplification, such as hearing aids, cochlear implants, and hearing assistive technology. If a flat configuration is present, for example, the audiologist selects a hearing aid with a flatter frequency response, whereas a high-frequency emphasis instrument is selected for a patient who demonstrates a sloping configuration. Audiogram configuration, in conjunction with knowledge regarding average conversational speech, may also play a role in referral for communication strategy training, speech and/or language therapy, parent-infant training, and other (re)habilitative strategies.

Symmetry

Symmetry, the last parameter discussed, compares magnitude and configuration of the right ear with that of the left ear. This characteristic is also often "eyeballed," as opposed to exactly quantified, and may vary from audiologist to audiologist. One useful clinical definition is to term the ears "symmetric" if AC thresholds of the right ear are within 10 dB of corresponding frequency's left ear AC thresholds. This determination provides the clinician with information regarding symmetry between ears during everyday listening and may also provide helpful information toward the rehabilitative process. For example, this information may be beneficial in determining need for binaural versus monaural amplification or whether preferential seating is in order. One must also consider comparison of each ear's BC thresholds when determining presence of symmetry. Unexplained asymmetry may be one indication of possible central pathology and may be cause for differential diagnosis referral.

IMPARTING PURE-TONE FINDINGS

Counseling is an integral aspect of the audiologist's responsibilities and one major area is to explain test results on completion of the audiogram. Skill and practice are necessary as the clinician learns to efficiently explain the pure-tone audiogram. The following is a sample explanation of audiometric findings. Vocabulary and communication style are geared toward individual patient needs, abilities, and communication skills.

> Here is a graph that provides a picture of your hearing, with the right ear recorded in red and the left ear recorded in blue. Across the top are the pitches of the tones you heard, from low to high as we move from left to right. Loudness levels are shown along the side, ranging from very soft at the top to very loud at the bottom. The "Os" represent softest levels you heard with the right ear earphone and the "Xs" represent the softest levels you heard with the left one.

The clinician then explains the magnitude of hearing loss, if present, in each ear and across the frequency range. The audiologist incorporates information about configuration, if the patient hears all pitches equally, or if the patient hears some more acutely than others. This is followed by an explanation of ear symmetry and bone conduction testing. It is helpful here to use an anatomic drawing of the ear as a counseling tool. The clinician explains that the "brackets" represent the softest level heard when the bone conduction vibrator was in place. A description of type of hearing loss follows, utilizing the anatomic chart to enhance explanation. Following explanation of the pure-tone audiogram, the audiologist explains speech audiometry, immittance and any other diagnostic findings. Finally, the clinician is prepared to counsel, answer questions, and make recommendations that initiate the roadmap toward remediation.

REFERENCES

Dobie, R. A., & Berlin, C. I. (1979). Influence of otitis media on hearing and development. *Annals of Otolaryngology, Rhinology, and Laryngology*, *88*(Suppl. 60), 48–53.

Skinner, M. W. (1978). The hearing of speech during language acquisition. *Otolaryngology Clinics of North America, 11*, 631–650.

Stach, B. A. (1998). *Clinical audiology: An introduction.* San Diego, CA: Singular.

6 *Masking*

MASKING IN THE HEARING SCIENCES

Masking is an important concept in the hearing sciences, and the student of Audiology must understand it from a broader, theoretical perspective prior to applying it to the clinical setting. Masking is defined as the interference in perception of a wanted signal caused by presence of another stimulus. In a listener's environment, there are countless daily instances where masking occurs: listening to someone talk from another room when the water is running, conversing in a restaurant with a friend when background music is present, or carrying on a conversation while walking by a construction site. The intended signal may take on many forms, such as music or conversation. Likewise, the masker that is interfering with the intended signal may take on many forms: one-talker speech stimuli, many-talker speech stimuli, various forms of noise, music, and others.

As one studies aspects of the masking process, it is important to consider frequency, intensity, and temporal aspects of both signal and masker. Many types of noise are emitted by a clinical audiometer, including white noise, speech noise, and narrow-band noise. The spectrum of white noise involves representation of all frequencies at equal amplitude, although there is dependence on the transducer used and often a diminished response above 6 kHz. The frequency response of speech noise is approximately 300 to 3000 Hz, or the most important frequencies for speech stimuli. Narrow-band noise

(NBN) is a white noise filtered into limited bandwidths (Studebaker, 1962). It is described in terms of its center frequency, its bandwidth of frequencies that are no more than 3 dB below the peak frequency, and rejection rate or decrease in intensity within octave intervals on each side of the band (Sanders, 1991). As one considers frequency aspects of both the signal and the masking noise, one notes that masking is most effective when the masker is of the same frequency spectrum as the intended stimulus. That is, if a clinician wishes to mask a 1 kHz pure-tone signal, the process will be most efficient when a narrow band of noise centered around 1 kHz is implemented. Differences in the effectiveness of masking occur when the signal and the masker are of differing frequency spectra. Masking may still be effective if the masker is of a lower frequency than the stimulus. If the masker is of a higher frequency than the stimulus, however, there will be a release from masking. That is, masking will not be as effective and the signal will more likely be heard. Examples of these phenomena are readily apparent when a clinician performs hearing screenings in a school and outside a sound suite. Most ambient noise within the school classrooms will likely be of a low frequency, such as may be found with heating and ventilation systems. As this ambient noise serves as a masker, hearing screening signals at 500 Hz may not be heard as effectively as the higher frequencies. Audiologists screen in these environments at 1 kHz, 2 kHz, and 4 kHz; these frequencies will be heard effectively, despite the ambient noise levels, although the higher frequencies may be easier to perceive. If trying to perceive a 1 kHz tone in the presence of a higher frequency noise, the listener will likely be successful.

The capability for a masker to be effective is also dependent on the intensity of the noise. If sufficient amplitude is not present, the noise may not effectively mask and the signal may still be perceived by the listener. Effective masking refers to just enough intensity so that the noise or masker effectively masks or interferes with the listener's perception of the signal. A critical bandwidth of noise is present, containing most of the energy necessary for performing the masking task. Energy outside this critical band contributes very little to the masking process (Hamill & Price, 2008).

Temporal aspects are also critical parameters related to the masking process, although listeners typically encounter simultaneous occurrence of the signal and masker. Backward masking occurs when the signal precedes the masker and the process is effective if the masker and stimulus are within 50 milliseconds of one another. Forward masking occurs when the masker precedes the stimulus and the process is effective if the masker and stimulus are within 75 to 100 milliseconds of one another. If the two stimuli are further apart in time, both will likely be perceived and masking will not occur (Yost, 2000).

CLINICAL MASKING

Clinical masking in audiology is one of the most difficult clinical concepts for the student of Audiology to master. One learns the theory and rules of application, with optimum learning taking place during actual hands-on experiences. As with many aspects of clinical diagnostic audiology including pure-tone testing, one may initially learn concepts and rules of application from textbooks and within the classroom. The second part of this dual process, however, is to carry over these concepts into the clinic, bridging from classroom to hands-on experiences with patients.

An optimum way to begin a clinical masking discussion is to progress step-by-step through testing of a hypothetical patient. Suppose an adult patient has just undergone neuro-otologic surgery for a left acoustic neuroma and the audiologist is performing the follow-up audiologic evaluation. Despite best intraoperative monitoring efforts, the tumor was situated such that the VIIIth nerve was compromised, leaving little or no residual hearing sensitivity in the left ear. In performing pure-tone testing, the audiologist first tests the better right ear via air conduction and this results in normal hearing sensitivity from 250 to 8000 Hz. As the audiologist tests the left ear, he or she does not note "no response at the limits of the audiometric equipment, at least under the unmasked condition." Rather, responses are seen within the moderate to moderately severe hearing loss range and are variable as a function of frequency.

This example highlights several concepts, including one of the first principles of masking theory whereby the signal reaches intensity sufficient enough to cross over from the test ear (TE) and be perceived by the nontest ear (NTE). Interaural attenuation (IA) is a term associated with clinical masking, referring to amount by which the signal is attenuated as it loses energy while traveling to the NTE. When performing the masking procedure, it is important to differentiate the TE from the NTE. In the above example, the right ear is serving as the NTE and the left ear is serving as the TE. A helpful mnemonic device is to consider that *n*oise is delivered to the *N*TE during clinical masking, with both beginning with "N." Additionally and alliteratively, the *t*one is delivered to the *T*E where *t*rue *t*hresholds are being obtained.

When crossover occurs during pure-tone audiometry, the NTE is perceiving tones that are being presented to the TE and the positive responses described in the above example represent responses from the better ear. When this occurs in the absence of masking, a "shadow curve" may be obtained on the audiogram. This is an audiogram pattern where the unmasked thresholds of the poorer TE mirror the thresholds of the better NTE because the NTE is actually perceiving the signal. Clinical masking involves presenting a noise via earphone to the NTE, so that the NTE does not perceive the test signal. With proper masking procedures, thresholds obtained in the TE are a true reflection of its sensitivity.

Progressing through the pure-tone audiologic evaluation with the acoustic neuroma patient, the audiologist also performs bone conduction testing. Results for the better right ear are also within normal limits from 250 to 4000 Hz and no significant ABGs are seen. The audiologist chooses to physically place the BC transducer on the left mastoid and perform unmasked BC testing on the poorer ear. When this occurs, there is a simultaneous stimulation of both cochleas and unmasked BC results for the left-side mirror those previously obtained for the right ear from 250 to 4000 Hz. When viewing unmasked results, the audiologist has no way of knowing if these BC thresholds for the poorer ear are true thresholds, or if they are merely a reflection of the better right ear. The audiologist must once again perform the masking procedure, this time when obtaining BC thresholds for the TE or poorer left ear while presenting noise to the NTE. In this manner and with proper masking, the NTE is excluded from the testing process and results obtained are a reflection solely of the test ear sensitivity.

In this example and without proper masking, the audiologist may underestimate magnitude of the TE hearing loss and may also misinterpret the type of hearing loss. One may easily see implications of these errors that include improper recommendations and remediation strategies, as well as inappropriate medical referrals. It is important for the audiologist to apply rules of when to mask by AC and BC, to learn proper types and intensity of masking noise levels, to record results properly, and to adapt the proper procedures for obtaining masked thresholds. Audiologists have traditionally utilized many different masking procedures. Although exposure to these various procedures may be challenging for the student, he or she should embrace this learning experience and devise a rationale for the development of his or her own preferred procedures.

MASKING THEORY

Cross-hearing occurs when the stimulus that is presented to the TE crosses over via bone conduction to the NTE. When the stimulus is presented via AC, the pathway may be represented by a classic diagram that demonstrates a dual process of traveling around the head by AC transducer leakage and through the bones of the skull by BC. With an AC signal, there is some attenuation or diminishing of intensity as the signal travels from one ear to the other. This is known as interaural attenuation (IA). The "interaural" component of the definition is straightforward, indicating that the signal progresses from one ear (TE) to the other (NTE). In the above example, a certainly intensity level was required to be present in the TE before it could be barely perceived as threshold in the NTE. Figure 6–1A demonstrates crossover, as may be seen during AC testing. Figure 6–1B demonstrates crossover, as may be seen during BC testing.

The intensity level at which cross-hearing in the opposite ear occurs will vary, depending on a number of factors. First, there is IA variance as a function of frequency. Second, IA varies from patient to patient depending on head size, skull thickness, and a host of other physiologic factors. Third, IA varies as a function of transducer type with crossing over seen earlier (less intensity) with supra-aural earphones than with insert receivers. IA studies have noted the following approximate ranges with TDH supra-aural earphones as a function of frequency (Chaiklin, 1967; Coles & Priede, 1970; Killion et al, 1985; Sklare & Denenberg, 1987):

250 Hz	500 Hz	1 kHz	2 kHz	4 kHz	8 kHz
44–80 dB	45–80 dB	40–80 dB	45–75 dB	45–85 dB	45–80 dB

When performing BC testing with mastoid placement, the signal immediately crosses over and stimulates the intact cochlea on the opposite side, although some audiologists have observed a slight degree of IA in the higher frequencies. When forehead BC placement is used, the signal stimulates both cochleas simultaneously. Because of the immediate crossing over, some clinicians advocate always utilizing masking during BC testing. One may readily see the importance of masking during BC testing, so that individual ear information and true thresholds are attained. When masking is performed during AC testing, noise is presented to the NTE via supra-

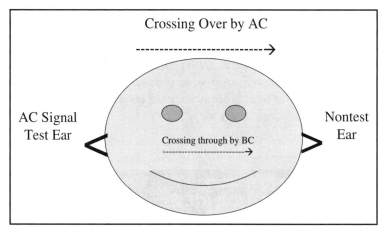

A

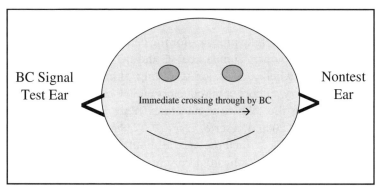

B

Figure 6–1. A. Crossover by air conduction **B.** Crossover by bone conduction.

aural or insert earphone. When masking is performed during BC testing, the BC oscillator is in place on the TE mastoid process or forehead while an earphone delivers the appropriate level of masking noise to the NTE.

Central masking is a phenomenon that occurs when the presence of a noise stimulus independently results in a threshold shift of approximately 5 dB, even though cross-hearing is not occurring (Liden et al., 1959; Zwislocki, 1953). This phenomenon is felt to be a function of the efferent central nervous system and may increase to a threshold shift of as great as 10 to 12 dB with greater intensity levels of noise (Studebaker, 1962).

RULES OF WHEN MASKING SHOULD BE IMPLEMENTED

Air Conduction (AC) Testing

The audiologist carefully prepares for the clinical masking situation. The examiner compares unmasked AC and BC results to apply the rule related to when to mask for AC testing. Although masking procedures may vary, authors of introductory audiology texts consistently advocate using the following guidelines (Katz & Lezynski, 2002; Martin & Clark, 2009; Roeser & Clark, 2007; Stach, 1998). Masking should be performed when the AC threshold of the TE exceeds the BC threshold of the NTE by 40 dB or greater. In determining which frequencies to mask in the TE, the audiologist is considering which are true thresholds and which could be a result of NTE participation. The rule is applied frequency by frequency, comparing each TE AC threshold with the corresponding NTE BC threshold. The need for masking is a frequency by frequency determination; masking may be performed at some frequencies and not at others. As a threshold is questioned, the clinician prepares to re-establish the TE threshold by introducing noise to the NTE via the masking process. Figure 6–2 shows an audiogram where masking is needed for AC thresholds of the right ear at 250 and 500 Hz.

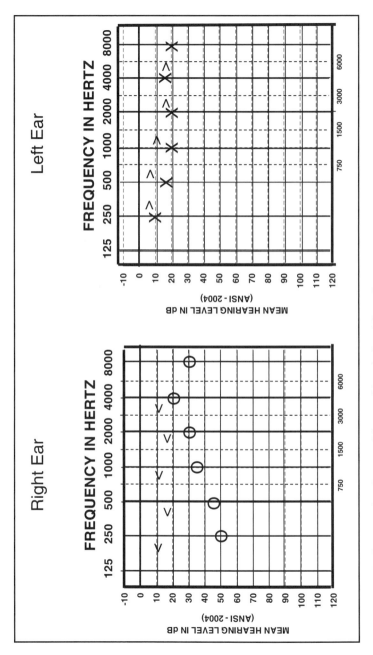

Figure 6–2. Audiogram showing need for masking during AC testing.

In examining the need to mask, one may question the rationale for a difference of 40 dB or more between the AC threshold of the TE and the BC threshold of the NTE. One must consider IA values and that they vary as a function of frequency, individual, and transducer. Although IA values may be greater than 40 dB, they have rarely been measured at less than 40 dB and it becomes cumbersome to measure cross-hearing for each individual patient as a function of frequency. Therefore, a conservative approach is followed and the criterion adopted by most clinicians is a 40 dB difference. One variation is that some audiologists apply this 40 dB rule at lower and middle frequencies, while applying a 45 dB rule at 2 kHz and a 50 dB rule at 4 kHz, and 8 kHz where IA values are greater (Goldstein & Newman, 1994). In applying a conservative approach with regard to the IA value, one may on occasion mask when masking is not needed; this engages few consequences and the audiologist will not be clinically overlooking important cases where masking should have taken place. Because IA values are higher when using insert earphones, in that the NTE does not participate as readily, some audiologists may adapt a higher value than with supra-aural earphones. IA ranges for inserts have been reported from 95 to 100 dB at 250 Hz, 85 to 95 dB at 500 Hz, 70 to 85 dB at 1 kHz, 70 to 75 dB at 2 kHz, 75 to 85 dB at 4 kHz, and 70 to 75 dB at 6 kHz (Killion et al., 1985; Konig, 1962; Roeser & Clark, 2007; Sklare & Denenberg, 1987). Although still conservative while using this transducer, some audiologists may mask when there is a 50 dB or greater difference between the AC threshold of the TE and the BC threshold of the NTE. Figure 6–3 demonstrates a simulated listener where masking is needed for the AC TE threshold because it is 40 dB or more poorer than the BC threshold of the NTE.

One may also question the rationale for comparing the AC threshold of one ear with the BC threshold of the other ear. As may be seen in Figure 6–1A, crossover occurs via AC and BC transduction during AC stimulus delivery; BC sensitivity is utilized for comparison

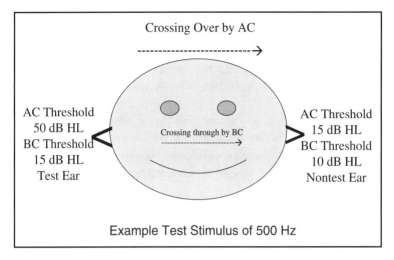

Figure 6–3. Head simulation showing need for masking during AC testing.

as it theoretically should be better than or equal to AC sensitivity and stimulation may occur here initially. The crucial concept is that the NTE will most probably respond sooner and more readily via BC than via AC. It might be noted that, in fact, almost all crossover occurs via bone conduction.

Students of Audiology may inquire about applying the AC rule to mask by comparing the AC threshold of the TE with the AC threshold of the NTE. If this rule is applied in a narrowly focused manner without considering the BC threshold, some thresholds may be missed that should be masked by not comparing to the BC threshold of the NTE. However, this AC to AC comparison could be a corollary of the primary rule if AC and BC are superimposed and the 40 dB difference also exists between AC (TE) and BC (NTE) as in Example A. In this case, the AC and BC thresholds of the right ear should be masked.

Example A:

	Right (TE)	**Left (NTE)**
AC threshold	40 dB HL	0 dB HL
BC threshold	0 dB HL	0 dB HL

One must exercise caution and utilize the primary rule, as opposed to the corollary when AC and BC are not superimposed as in Example B. If AC of the TE were compared with AC of the NTE in this example, masking may be determined as unnecessary when it should be performed:

Example B:

	Right (TE)	**Left (NTE)**
AC threshold	40 dB HL	20 dB HL
BC threshold	0 dB HL	0 dB HL

One viable way for students of Audiology to learn appropriate masking procedures is to obtain all AC and BC unmasked thresholds prior to applying rules of when to mask. The student may then compare AC thresholds of the right ear to BC thresholds of the left ear in a frequency by frequency manner. The left ear may then become the TE, as the student applies rules and compares its AC thresholds to BC thresholds of the opposite ear in a frequency by frequency manner. As the audiologist carries classroom knowledge into the clinical situation, these procedures may be adapted and streamlined without forfeiting accuracy. For example, an AC threshold of the TE may be compared with a best BC threshold at a specific frequency regardless of ear, to determine presence of a true threshold and need for masking. Most clinicians perform AC testing before performing BC testing and may mask as they proceed through obtaining AC thresholds, exercising expertise and clinical insight in determining if masking is necessary.

Bone Conduction (BC) Testing

BC thresholds are typically obtained after AC testing and should be masked any time a significant air-bone gap (ABG) exists in the TE. A significant ABG exists at any frequency when the AC threshold of the TE exceeds the BC threshold of the TE by greater than 10 dB. Some audiologists consider a significant ABG to be a 10 dB or greater difference between AC and BC thresholds. Some clinicians feel it is necessary to mask all BC thresholds because BC stimuli immediately cross over to the opposite cochlea when presented to one cochlea. Although this is an excellent thought, it may not be clinically relevant to determine exact magnitude of ABGs, particularly if the examiner has already ascertained that they are not significant. Presence or absence of significant ABGs on the audiogram are utilized to help determine type of hearing impairment. The testing session may become overly laborious if masking is implemented unnecessarily while obtaining all BC thresholds on every patient. Example C below demonstrates AC and BC thresholds that have been obtained at 2 kHz for each ear. Although masking is not necessary for AC thresholds, there are significant ABGs in both ears and each BC threshold must be masked. That is, the right BC threshold must be reestablished under the masked condition with noise presented to the left ear as the NTE and the left ear threshold must be re-established under the masked condition with noise presented to the right ear as the NTE.

Example C:

	Right Ear	**Left Ear**
AC threshold	30 dB HL	25 dB HL
BC threshold	5 dB HL	10 dB HL

Audiologists who choose to perform BC testing via forehead placement find that they may always set up their patients for masking. That is, they place the BC oscillator on the forehead and then place inserts or other earphones for delivery of masking noise in the NTE. The occlusion effect remains a constant entity as ear canals are occluded during unmasked and masked BC testing. The audiologist does not have to physically enter the sound suite, interrupt the session, and replace the BC vibrator and masking earphone as he or she prepares to test the other ear. The audiologist may proceed accurately and efficiently through the session, even if he or she wishes to mask each BC threshold.

TYPE OF NOISE USED CLINICALLY

As clinical masking is performed, a dual-channel audiometer is in order such that the pure-tone stimulus may be presented to the TE while narrow-band noise is presented to the NTE. Historically, audiometers were accompanied by noise generators where center frequency of noise had to be manually changed to correspond to the frequency of the pure tone. With current technology, the narrow-band noise automatically changes with pure-tone stimulus frequency. Noise levels historically also had to be biologically calibrated according to effective masking, or the intensity level necessary to just mask the tone and today these levels are automatically incorporated into audiometric equipment.

As the audiologist learns while studying the hearing sciences, the most effective masker of a pure-tone stimulus is a noise composed of the same frequency. For this reason, narrow bands of noise (NBN) are utilized in the NTE during clinical masking of AC and BC thresholds. A line spectrum of simple harmonic motion involves frequency displayed across the x-axis from lower to higher and amplitude shown along the y-axis from softer upward to louder. Only one frequency, the test frequency, is represented. The spectrum of the narrow band of noise corresponding to that pure-tone stimulus also is very narrowly centered about that same test frequency.

AC diagnostic measures other than pure-tone audiometry may be performed in the audiology clinic and the same rules regarding "when to mask" for such procedures are similar to those already discussed for AC pure-tone testing. These rules should serve as a guide regarding when the NTE may be participating and when it becomes necessary to keep the NTE occupied with masking noise presentation. Similarly, pure-tone stimuli may be the stimuli of choice in performing diagnostic measures other than pure-tone threshold audiometry. When masking is performed for such procedures as tonal stimuli are presented to the TE, the clinician chooses to present NBN to the NTE.

Although speech audiometry is beyond the scope of this textbook, one may recall that the spectrum of speech stimuli encompasses many frequencies and many intensities as a function of frequency. This is in contrast to the narrow pure-tone stimulus spectrum. The audiologist applies masking rules when performing speech audiometry to make certain that the NTE is not participating in the testing session. When masking is in order, speech noise (SN) is most often the noise of choice to be presented to the NTE. The spectrum of SN involves a much wider band of frequencies and those frequencies are often referred to as the important frequencies composing the average conversational speech spectra.

PLATEAU

Once the audiologist determines a need for masking, the masking procedure is initiated. A two-channel audiometer is in order, with the pure-tone stimulus delivered via one channel and the NBN delivered via the second channel. With AC testing, the signal is delivered via one supra-aural or insert earphone to the TE while the noise is delivered via the other earphone to the NTE. The audiologist may either obtain masked thresholds as he or she progresses through pure-tone testing or after obtaining all unmasked thresholds. The audiologist instructs the patient that he or she will be hearing a noise in the designated ear, sounding like static. The patient is to ignore the noise and to raise a hand or otherwise respond each time the tone is heard, even if very soft. The clinician reiterates that this is the task that the listener has been performing during pure-tone audiometry, other than hearing a noise that will be presented to the NTE. Patients will often respond to the noise on its presentation and must be reinstructed to respond only to the tone, while ignoring the noise. With BC testing, the signal is delivered via the bone conduction oscillator to the TE while the noise is delivered to the NTE via supra-aural or insert earphone. If supra-aural earphones are used, the unused earphone may rest at the top of the head. Instructions are the same as described for AC. The patient should be instructed to respond to the tone, even if he or she feels it is not perceived in the TE. Furthermore, he should be instructed that the extra earphone is not meant to cover the test ear. As previously discussed, some audiologists prefer a BC vibrator forehead placement with inserts in place to deliver noise to the NTE during the masking procedure.

There are many correct masking procedures available to the clinical audiologist and many formulae to determine initial intensity level of noise to present to the NTE. Prior to discussion of more popular methods, definitions and additional theoretical insights are in order. Figure 6–4 demonstrates representation of a classic diagram that appears in the masking literature and helps the student of Audiology understand underlying masking theory.

One notes presentation level of the NBN on the abscissa in dB HL and presentation level of the pure-tone stimuli on the ordinate in dB HL. This graph depicts several very important definitions that are crucial toward the understanding of masking concepts, with points on the graph representing patient responses. The first definition is undermasking and is represented on the graph as the segment from A to B. This segment represents the intensity level of noise that may be presented, but is not sufficiently intense to mask the tone in the

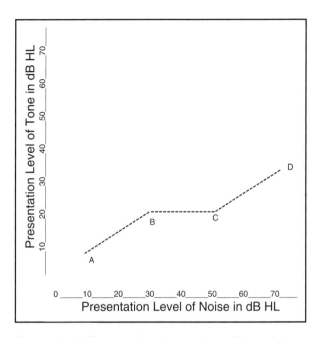

Figure 6–4. Diagram showing undermasking, plateau, and overmasking.

NTE. When one considers the phenomenon of crossing over from the TE to NTE, this situation represents an insufficient intensity level of masking noise presented to the NTE. The tonal stimulus is still crossing over from the TE to the NTE and is being perceived by the NTE; the NTE is participating in testing and true thresholds are not obtained in the TE because there is not enough noise to mask the signal. With effective masking (segment B-C), there is a sufficient intensity level of noise, such that the tone is effectively masked and the proper procedure is performed. With implementation of effective masking, the NTE ear does not participate in the testing and thresholds obtained in the TE are accurate ones. Segment B-C on the graph shown in Figure 6-4 shows a range of effective masking.

There is a range or plateau of NBN intensity whereby masking is effective. Location B represents a minimum effective noise level of masking. This is the minimum intensity level of noise at which accurate masking occurs and true thresholds may be obtained. Location C represents a maximum effective noise level of masking, defined as the maximum intensity level of noise at which accurate masking may occur and true thresholds may be obtained. One may readily see several important points here. The first is that the formulae to express how much initial NBN to present are very precise, are individualized for each patient, and have been carefully constructed according to complex masking theory. It is not sufficient to just "guestimate" an initial noise level or for the audiologist to "toss in a constant level of noise" for all patients without proper justification and careful consideration. The second important point is that masked pure-tone thresholds must be maintained over a range or plateau of noise before they may be accepted and recorded. It is not sufficient to note that a patient responded positively to a tone presented within a certain, single level of noise; rather, the patient must respond positively to the tone over several levels of noise. The audiologist must exercise caution, making certain that the masking noise is intense enough for masking to occur, that it is not too soft, and that it is not too loud.

As one studies the graph in Figure 6–4, one notes that the A–B undermasking segment is linear and progresses from left to right at an approximate 45-degree angle. That is, a certain increment in the noise level leads to a corresponding and equivalent increment in the tonal presentation level at which the patient responds. The same linear increase may be observed in segment C–D that represents overmasking and the graph again progresses upward from left to right at an approximate 45-degree angle. Section B–C is flat and is a section of major importance, in that masking is effectively occurring within this area. When masking is effectively being performed and a plateau reached, the listener hears the tone at the same dB HL level while the noise is increased by several increments. These incremental increases of noise, where patient responses are consistent at one test signal presentation level, represent the plateau.

Section C-D of Figure 6-4 shows the area of overmasking, where the noise is too loud for the masking process to be efficiently performed and for true thresholds to be obtained. If one visualizes a diagram of the head and recalls the previous IA discussion, one may note that crossing over to the opposite ear is occurring in this situation. This time, however, the masking noise presented to the NTE is too loud, is crossing over to the TE, and is interfering with perception of the tone in the TE. In this case, true thresholds are not being obtained.

The plateau method of masking process was first described by Hood in 1960. Although other procedures are and have been utilized toward the masking procedure, the plateau method is one time honored and classic approach that is widely accepted within many audiology clinics. Its effectiveness is worth time exerted and plateau procedures become quick and efficient for the audiologist, as he or she gains practice and experience.

As audiologists implement the plateau method of masking, they may utilize a variety of formulae for determining intensity level of NBN to initially present in the NTE. Many viable formulae exist, although all examiners share the common goal of reaching effective masking levels and a plateau of masking noise. Furthermore, all examiners share the common goal of obtaining true thresholds in the TE while introducing masking noise to the NTE. An analogy to help the student, who may be confused by numerous formulae and masking procedures recommended by clinical preceptors, is as follows. As one yet again views the B-C section of Figure 6-4, one may note that this area represents the clinician's goal or final destination. That is, all clinicians are striving toward accurate masked thresholds that have been attained through effective masking procedures. The analogy lies in viewing section B-C as a desired location to which all clinicians are traveling. Many points along section A-B represent the various beginning intensity levels, presented on initiating the masking procedure. The clinician starts at an undermasking level and works toward effective masking, with the various available formulae dictating the many points along this A–B section. In furthering the analogy, these might represent many different subway stations and starting points that are moving in the same direction and toward the shared goal, as clinicians work their way toward the ultimate outcome or destination outlined above.

When determining the intensity level of noise to initially present to the NTE, most formulae begin with consideration of the AC pure-tone threshold of the NTE at the test frequency. Recall that the masking noise is presented via AC to the NTE, whether the stimuli presented to the TE are via AC or BC. Although the masking process is complex, it becomes simplified with thought and reasoning; it would make little sense to present a tone to the NTE that is subaudible or softer than the AC threshold for that ear. Many audiologists may add a constant to that, such as 10 dB, so that the noise is not presented exactly at threshold. This also may reduce some time from the plateau-obtaining procedure, by starting at a slightly higher level of masking noise. Finally, some audiologists may add the magnitude of any ABG at the test frequency in the NTE. One recommended formula for determining starting intensity level of noise in the NTE then contains three components and becomes: AC threshold of the NTE plus 10 dB constant plus ABG (NTE). The masking mastering process involves learning such procedures and formulae, applying these guidelines to the actual audiogram, and then implementing clinically with the patient. With experience, this process becomes streamlined. Figure 6–5 shows an audiogram where masking is needed for the AC threshold at 250 Hz. That is, this threshold is questioned because of crossover and the masking procedure must be initiated with noise presented to the NTE. The amount of noise initially presented to the NTE to re-establish this threshold is as follows. In this case, a narrow band of noise centered around 250 Hz is delivered to the left ear, which is the NTE. The initial NBN presentation level, according to one of many accepted formulae, is 10 dB (AC threshold of NTE at 250 Hz) plus 10 dB constant plus 5 dB (ABG at 250 Hz in the NTE) equals 25 dB HL.

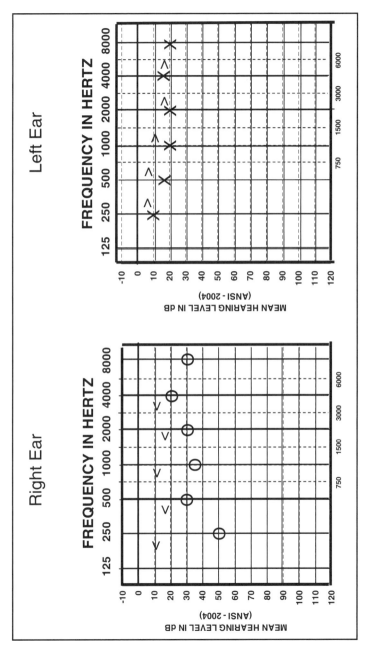

Figure 6–5. Audiogram where AC and BC masking are needed, demonstrating noise intensity levels.

When one applies the rules of masking for the audiogram in Figure 6-5, one may see that significant ABGs exist for the right ear at all frequencies except 4 KHz. For the left ear, no significant ABGs are noted and, therefore, masking is not necessary. In preparing the patient for masking, the BC oscillator remains on the right TE and an earphone is placed on the left NTE. The audiologist prepares to re-establish thresholds in the right ear from 250 to 4000 Hz while presenting noise to the left. As previously discussed, an alternative method is to mask all instances where ABGs of 10 dB or greater exist with mastoid placement. A third method is to utilize forehead placement and to mask all BC thresholds, presenting noise to the NTE.

There are numerous formulae to determine initial noise presentation levels when masking BC thresholds. A common rule begins with the AC threshold of the NTE as a base, because the noise is presented to that ear via AC. Many audiologists also add a constant of approximately 10 dB, the rationale for and advantages of which have been previously discussed. Many clinicians then add the occlusion effect (OE), a phenomenon that occurs primarily with lower frequency stimuli. The occlusion effect is a perceived improvement in BC hearing, measured following occlusion of the ear canal. Recall that unmasked BC thresholds are often obtained without presence of an earphone; when the patient is set up for masking, there is earphone placement on the NTE and the OE may be seen prior to presentation of noise. The audiologist may establish this value on each individual patient and may add the improvement from unoccluded to occluded condition to the masking formula. Certainly, there are advantages to calculating the OE for each individual patient as opposed to utilizing average values for each and every patient. An alternative is to add average OE values, although OE values vary widely from patient to patient and an individual's OE may be very different from the average value. Average values accumulated from previous studies are approximately 21 dB at 250 Hz, 18 dB at 500 Hz, and 7 dB at 1 kHz (Roeser & Clark, 2007). Because audiologists test in 5 dB increments, recommended average values for formula incorporation might be 20 dB at 250 Hz, 20 dB at 500 Hz, and 5 dB at 1 kHz. If using this one of many formulae, the following initial intensity levels of noise would be implemented in the NTE (see Figure 6–5 audiogram) as the audiologist begins the BC masking process:

250 Hz: 10 dB (AC threshold of NTE) + 10 dB + OE (individual or average value)

500 Hz: 15 dB (AC threshold of NTE) + 10 dB + OE (individual or average value)

1 kHz: 20 dB (AC threshold of NTE) + 10 dB + OE (individual or average value)

2 kHz: 20 dB (AC threshold of NTE) + 10 dB + OE (individual or average value)

MASKING PROCEDURE

The actual masking procedure is the same for AC and BC. With AC testing, the appropriate rule is applied to determine necessity and instructions are provided to the patient. Following instructions, the unmasked threshold is re-established at the desired frequency in the TE, in the absence of noise. The appropriate intensity level of noise is presented, as determined by preferred formula, in a continuously-on manner to the NTE. The modified Hughson-Westlake procedure is not initiated. Rather, the audiologist re-presents the tone at the unmasked threshold level in the presence of noise. Whenever there is a positive response to the tone, the audiologist raises the noise level by 5 dB. The audiologist then re-presents the tone amidst this new and higher level of noise. Whenever there is no response, the tone is raised by 5 dB and is re-presented. The audiologist manipulates controls of the two-channel audiometer in this manner, gradually increasing stimulus and noise in 5 dB steps according to patient response. In this manner, the audiologist either embarks on the initial ascending or the flattened portion of the plateau graph shown in Figure 6-4. The goal is to present the tone and elicit positive responses at a constant intensity level while the noise is raised three times in 5 dB increments, achieving a plateau of 15 dB. Audiologists may vary with regard to the magnitude of plateau that they wish to achieve and will accept for demonstrating threshold. Although a 15 dB plateau may be ideal, it may become necessary to accept and record thresholds obtained via a 10 dB plateau. An example of this process appears below, resulting in a masked AC threshold at 4 kHz:

	RE (TE)	**LE (NTE)**	**Response**
Intensity level	40 dB HL	unmasked	+
	40 dB HL	20 dB HL	−
	45 dB HL	20 dB HL	+
	45 dB HL	25 dB HL	+
	45 dB HL	30 dB HL	+
	45 dB HL	35 dB HL	+

In this case, the initial noise level presented to the NTE was determined by a preferred formula, taking into consideration the AC threshold of that ear. On delivery of noise, the patient did not hear the stimulus at the original unmasked threshold level. The tonal level therefore, was raised by 5 dB and a positive response was elicited. As there was a positive response, the noise was raised by 5 dB and this process continued. The audiologist was able to raise the noise in 5 dB increments for an overall plateau of 15 dB, while the patient maintained hearing the tone in the TE. The masked AC threshold is 45 dB HL. It is important to record noise levels on the audiogram, from lower to upper limit of the plateau. In this case, the audiologist would record a 20/35 dB plateau. That is, the patient responded positively to the tone at 45 dB HL over noise increments from 20 to 25 dB HL, 25 to 30 dB HL, and 30 to 35 dB HL.

The procedure for BC is similar, other than placement of the BC oscillator over the TE mastoid and placement of an earphone over the NTE. Recall that some audiologists prefer mastoid placement whereas others prefer forehead placement. Instructions are the same as for AC and have been previously described. The unmasked threshold is re-established via BC oscillator with earphone in place on the NTE, in the absence of noise. Recall that the occlusion effect (OE) may have an effect on this perceived unmasked threshold at lower to mid frequencies, merely by placement of the earphone. The initial noise level is presented in a continuously-on fashion, according to the audiologist's preferred formula for determining narrow-band noise intensity level. Whenever there is a positive response to the tonal stimulus, the noise is raised by 5 dB. Whenever the patient does not respond to the tone at a specific level, the tone is raised in a 5 dB increment. This alternative tone-raising by 5 dB and noise-raising by 5 dB process continues with use of the dual-channel audiometer until plateau is reached. The audiologist has determined threshold when a positive response to the tone is maintained over three 5 dB increments of noise intensity, or a plateau of 15 dB.

Katz and Lezynski (2002) have described a step procedure that may be used to minimize masking steps, especially if the audiologist finds the plateau method cumbersome. This procedure is based on Effective Masking Level (EML), defined as the level to which a masking noise raises threshold in the NTE. For example, 40 dB EML will shift threshold to 40 dB HL if thresholds are initially 40 dB HL or better. During the step-masking process, Initial Masking (IM) is presented to the NTE. The presentation level must be intense enough to shift threshold without the occurrence of overmasking. On re-establishing threshold in the presence of the IM level, the clinician gains immediate insight regarding presence of crossover to the NTE. Although calculation of IM levels vary according to clinician

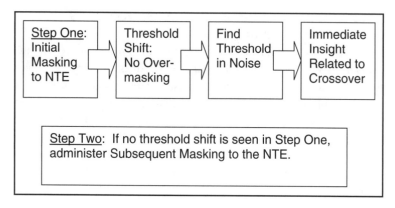

Figure 6–6. The step procedure for masking.

preference, the authors recommend that 30 dB EML above the AC threshold of the NTE be utilized.

Often, there will be no shift in threshold in the presence of masking noise or the threshold shift will be minimal (5–10 dB). As a second step to the process, the authors recommend implementing Subsequent Masking (SM) if the threshold shift in the presence of IM is 20 dB or more. As with IM levels, SM levels must be determined such that overmasking does not occur. Although clinician variability is wide, the authors recommend presentation of an additional +20 dB SL (re: EML) when additional masking noise is needed during the second step of the process. Figure 6-6 demonstrates a block diagram of the step procedure.

RECORDING OF RESULTS

When the audiologist performs masking of AC thresholds, there are three major outcomes that could occur. The first is that the masked threshold may be the same as the unmasked threshold. The masking process is necessary to verify that this is the case. The second outcome is that, following the masking procedure, there could be no response at the limits of the audiometric equipment at that particular frequency. Third, the AC response could fall somewhere in between the first two options (unmasked threshold and limit of the equipment). Once masking has taken place, the appropriate masked symbol should be recorded on the audiogram, as discussed in Chapter 4. Unmasked thresholds should be removed as they are no longer valid. Valid AC thresholds (whether masked or unmasked as a function of frequency) should be connected by straight lines on the audiogram, and the clinician always should be aware of neatness and uniformity of symbols. The noise levels also should be recorded, often just below that frequency line on the audiogram, from lowest to highest point of plateau attained. Implementation of accurate masking techniques will help ensure that appropriate interpretations are made regarding magnitude and other parameters of hearing impairment.

When the audiologist performs masking during BC testing, there are also three major outcomes that may occur. The first is that the masked threshold may be equivalent to the unmasked threshold. It is necessary, of course, to perform the masking procedure to verify this outcome. The second outcome is that the masked BC threshold could fall to meet the AC threshold. If there is no usable hearing, there could be no response at the limits of the audiometric equipment. Recall that limits of equipment are met at lower intensity levels with BC stimuli than with AC stimuli, due to equipment limitations. The proper symbol should be recorded, denoting the masked BC threshold displaying an arrow, to signify that the limits were reached. Third, the response could fall somewhere between the first two options: between the unmasked BC threshold and the AC threshold. The appropriate masked BC threshold symbol should be recorded on the audiogram, with its corresponding unmasked thresholds eradicated. Neatness continues to be imperative and the plateau of noise once again should be recorded, often below the appropriate frequency line of the audiogram. One may see that obtaining accurate masked thresholds is critical for comparison of air-bone relationships and determination of hearing loss type. If errors are made regarding type of hearing loss, serious remediation strategy consequences may occur, such as referring for medical management when unnecessary or improper amplification selection.

SENSORINEURAL ACUITY LEVEL (SAL) TEST

The Sensorineural Acuity Level (SAL) test is an older measure that has been utilized to help estimate the magnitude of air-bone gaps (ABGs) and conductive component of a hearing loss (Jerger & Tillman, 1960). The test may be especially helpful diagnostically when traditional bone conduction testing may not be performed, especially in instances where clinical masking is in order. Examples of such instances may be with pediatric patients unable to perform "traditional masking tasks," cases where masked results are questionable/unattainable via more traditional protocols, and estimation of smaller-sized ABGs.

The SAL test is performed by presenting noise through the bone conduction vibrator and pure-tone stimuli through the earphones of the audiometer. This protocol is opposite of more standard procedures whereby noise is delivered through the earphones and pure-tone stimuli through the bone conduction vibrator. The first step in performing the test is to ascertain the AC threshold via earphone at a certain frequency and in the ear of choice (Stach, 1998, pp. 225–227). The clinician then delivers narrow-band noise (NBN) centered at the test frequency, at its maximum level of intensity. The third step is to reestablish the AC threshold, accomplished in the first step, this time in the presence of noise. The audiologist then calculates the level of threshold shift, if any, in dB HL. It should be noted that the SAL test may also be performed with use of speech stimuli and this may be especially beneficial with evaluation of children.

Before a clinician performs the SAL test, he or she establishes normative data with as many normally hearing listeners as possible. The normative data provide information about the extent of threshold shift with normal listeners, so that patient values may be compared to these norms. An equivalent shift should be seen if there is no hearing disorder at the cochlear level. As cochlear function is intact with both normal listeners and those with conductive hearing loss, the shift should be comparable. The first step is to ascertain the maximum narrow-band noise level for each frequency that may be tested. This is performed by placing the bone conduction vibrator on the forehead and increasing the narrow band of noise until a vibratory sensation is felt. The maximum NBN level for each frequency is recorded as that which occurs just prior to the vibratory sensation. With each of the normative subjects, AC pure-tone threshold is obtained at 1 kHz. Threshold is re-established in the presence of the maximum NBN level, with the noise presented via BC vibrator forehead placement. The difference between threshold in quiet and threshold in noise is the SAL norm. Normative data are collected for each frequency for each subject, with average values as a function of frequency utilized as the clinic normative value.

If no threshold shift is present, the audiologist may interpret the hearing loss as being sensorineural in type. This is because the cochlear disorder does not allow for perception of the noise or for the noise to interfere with perception of the tone. The threshold will shift if the hearing loss is conductive in type because the intact cochlea perceives the noise, with the noise serving to mask the patient's ability to hear the tone. In this case, the amount of shift may help to estimate the extent of the ABG at that frequency and in that ear.

Examples are provided below for a sensorineural hearing loss (A) and for a conductive hearing loss (B). The stimuli are a 2-kHz tone and corresponding narrow-band noise value, for illustration purposes:

Example A:

AC threshold in quiet = 30 dB HL

AC threshold in noise = 30 dB HL (performed in maximum BC noise)

SAL normative data = 35 dB HL

Conductive component = None

Example B:

AC threshold in quiet = 30 dB HL

AC threshold in noise = 50 dB HL (performed in maximum BC noise)

SAL normative data = 35 dB HL

Conductive component = 15 dB HL

SAL normative values, of course, will vary from clinic to clinic and from frequency to frequency. Similarly, the maximum BC Levels will also vary as a function of clinical facility and frequency.

CHALLENGING MASKING CASES

Pure-tone audiometry, including the masking process, involves behavioral measures that require some type of voluntary and subjective patient response. The masking task may be especially challenging for some patients, in that they must continue to listen for a very soft tone that is embedded within noise. Furthermore, they must disregard the noise presented to the NTE as they focus on hearing the very soft stimulus presented to the TE. Clinical masking is especially difficult with young children, the cognitively impaired, the developmentally disabled, individuals who require interpreter services in a native language, and other populations.

It may not be possible to obtain a plateau in some cases. For example, equipment limits of the masking noise may be reached before a plateau is noted. In the case of no plateau, the audiologist should reinstruct and repeat the attempt at obtaining masked threshold. If plateau again may not be reached, the attempt and outcome should be recorded on the audiogram. The audiologist may also achieve a plateau during testing that is less than or lower than the desired plateau range; for example, the audiologist may only achieve a 10 dB plateau when he or she typically attempts to obtain a 15 dB plateau. In these cases, the audiologist should also repeat the procedure and record results accurately, so that the audiogram viewer is aware that proper masking techniques were attempted.

Occasionally, the magnitude and type of hearing loss preclude standard and accurate masking techniques, creating a "masking dilemma" for audiologists. A classic example is presented by the patient exhibiting a moderate conductive hearing loss, bilaterally. One may easily visualize significant ABGs bilaterally, where one must mask all AC and BC thresholds of both ears. As one utilizes existing formulae to determine masking noise levels to present to the NTE, one considers the AC threshold of the NTE. As the clinician adjusts the level of NBN to accommodate the NTE AC threshold, concerns immediately may arise concerning crossover to the normal BC thresholds of the TE and interference with testing. Yet another example of a difficult masking case is where there is a large asymmetry in AC thresholds on the audiogram. Often, one may easily place masking noise into the better NTE, if indicated; however, if an ABG exists in the better ear and noise must be placed into the poorer NTE, overmasking could occur. Depending on the magnitude of hearing loss in the NTE, one may also reach the NBN limits of the equipment prior to obtaining plateau.

Although pure-tone audiometry including appropriate masking is a crucial foundation of the audiologic diagnostic battery, one must bear in mind that this testing is usually performed in conjunction with other tests. The audiologist learns that the various measures all provide important "pieces of the puzzle" and these pieces also serve as a system of cross-check for one other. When masking may not be performed or when results may be questionable, the audiologist may implement the tuning fork tests described in Chapter 7 as one way to verify results. Contributions to the verification process may be made in myriad other ways, such as through case history, medical and physical examination, and otoscopic examination. Type of hearing impairment and validity of significant ABGs may be validated via tympanometry and its provision of important information regarding middle ear status. Also within the immittance test battery, acoustic reflex thresholds may help to verify magnitude of hearing loss and the status of acoustic reflex arc components. Results of speech audiometry may also provide clues, as the audiologist exercises clinical insights in anticipating certain speech audiometric results in light of pure-tone findings. Some challenging populations may adapt to speech audiometry and accompanying masking techniques prior to adapting to those for pure-tone audiometry. In many cases, valid speech audiometric results may shed valuable clinical light on validity of results obtained during pure-tone testing. Electrophysiologic measures, such as Auditory Brainstem Response (ABR) testing, may also contribute valuable diagnostic information; for example, important clues may be provided regarding severity and type of hearing impairment, when masking may not be adequately performed.

The masking process is an extremely important component of pure-tone audiometry, presenting challenges for the student of Audiology and the experienced clinician. If not performed correctly, clinical errors could result such as misrepresentation of hearing loss type or magnitude. During the learning process, the audiologist first studies masking from a hearing science perspective, as well as various types and characteristics of masking noise. Study of clinical masking addresses theory and the need to rule out NTE participation, thereby helping to answer questions related to why masking is necessary. The audiologist progresses to viewing audiometric configurations and determining when masking is necessary via AC and BC testing and when performing other diagnostic measures. Further important questions to address involve exploration of various formulae to determine presentation levels of masking noise, with avoidance of both undermasking and overmasking. Finally, the clinician implements the masking procedure, knowing when to increase the stimulus level, when to increase the noise level, and when plateau has been reached. Recording of masked thresholds and noise levels is critical, as is interpretation of the masked pure-tone audiogram as an important piece of the larger diagnostic battery. Students successfully learn difficult masking techniques through application of academic principles to the actual clinical setting, implementation of techniques offered by knowledgeable mentors, and extensive practice.

REFERENCES

Chaiklin, J. B. (1967). Interaural attenuation and cross-hearing in air conduction audiometry. *Journal of Auditory Research, 7,* 413–424.

Coles, R. R. A., & Priede, V. M. (1970). On the misdiagnosis resulting from incorrect use of masking. *Journal of Laryngology and Otology, 84,* 41–63.

Goldstein, B. A., & Newman, C. W. (1994). Clinical masking: A decision-making process. In J. Katz (Ed.), *Handbook of clinical audiology* (pp. 109–131). Baltimore: Lippincott Williams & Wilkins.

Hamill, T. A., & Price, L. L. (2008). *The hearing sciences.* San Diego, CA: Plural.

Hood, J. D. (1960). The principles and practice of bone conduction audiometry: A review of the present position. *Laryngoscope, 70,* 1211–1228.

Jerger, J., & Tillman, T. (1960). A new method for clinical determination of sensorineural acuity level (SAL). *Archives of Otolaryngology, 71,* 948–953.

Katz, J. A., & Lezynski, J. (2002). Clinical masking. In J. A. Katz (Ed.), *Handbook of clinical audiology* (5th ed., pp. 124–141). Philadelphia: Lippincott Williams & Wilkins.

Killion, M. C., Wilber, L. A., & Gudmundson, G. I. (1985). Insert earphones for more interaural attenuation. *Hearing Instruments, 36*(2), 34–38.

Konig, E. (1962). On the use of hearing aid type earphones in clinical audiometry. *Acta Otolaryngologica, 55*, 331–341.

Liden, G., Nilsson, G., & Anderson, H. (1959). Masking in clinical audiometry. *Acta Oto-Laryngologica, 50*, 125–136.

Martin, F. N., & Clark, J. G. (2009). *Introduction to audiology* (10th ed.). Boston: Pearson.

Roeser, R. J., & Clark, J. L. (2007). Clinical masking. In R. J. Roeser, M. Valente, & H. Hosford-Dunn (Eds.), *Audiology diagnosis* (2nd ed., pp. 261–287). New York: Thieme Medical.

Sanders, J. A. (1991). Clinical masking. In W. F. Rintelmann (Ed.), *Hearing assessment* (2nd ed., pp. 1–38). Austin, TX: Pro-Ed.

Sklare, D. A., & Denenberg, L. J. (1987). Interaural attenuation for Tubephone insert earphones. *Ear and Hearing, 8*, 298–300.

Stach, B. A. (1998). *Clinical audiology: An introduction*. San Diego, CA: Singular.

Studebaker, G. A. (1962). On masking in bone-conduction testing. *Journal of Speech and Hearing Research, 5*, 215–227.

Yost, W. A. (2000). *Fundamentals of hearing: An introduction* (4th ed.). San Diego, CA: Academic Press.

Zwislocki, J. (1953). Acoustic attenuation between ears. *Journal of the Acoustical Society of America, 25*, 752–759.

7 *Unconventional Pure-Tone Techniques*

There are some patients with whom conventional techniques may not be performed or may not be optimal. These include infants and small children, developmentally delayed patients, cognitively impaired patients, patients who exaggerate hearing loss, and patients who undergo ototoxic monitoring.

THE PEDIATRIC PATIENT

With the advent of universal hearing screening, early identification of hearing impairment and an explosion of technology, the audiologist is capable of diagnosing hearing impairment at or shortly after birth. The sooner identification takes place, the earlier intervention strategies may be initiated.

Electrophysiology

Conventional techniques are subjective and behavioral ones, requiring some type of patient response such as raising a hand or pushing a button. In contrast, there are numerous physiologic/electrophysiologic measures that are objective and are utilized to estimate hearing threshold. These objective measures are performed through use of sophisticated, computerized equipment. Two different physiologic/ electrophysiologic measures are utilized for screening hearing of newborns and young infants under the approximate developmental age of six months: otoacoustic emissions (OAEs) and auditory brainstem response (ABR) testing. Pure-tone stimuli in the form of very short tone-bursts may be utilized to evoke both the ABR and the OAE waveforms. A second use of both OAEs and ABRs is toward differential neuro-otologic diagnosis and helping to determine integrity of anatomic and physiologic systems. Although originally devised for estimation of hearing threshold, clinical applications of such electrophysiologic measures have evolved toward differential diagnosis and site of lesion determination.

The complementary nature of the two measures is readily apparent, when one views a present ABR tracing as representing an intact peripheral hearing mechanism and lower brainstem (Goldstein & Aldrich, 1999). OAEs, on the other hand, represent responses originating from normal, healthy outer hair cells of the inner ear (Kemp, 1979).

Behavioral Observation Audiometry (BOA)

Especially prior to the advent of electrophysiologic measures, audiologists have utilized behavioral observation audiometry techniques (BOA) for testing children at a developmental age of approximately six months or younger. Calibrated stimuli, according to frequency and intensity parameters, are presented through sound suite loudspeakers, especially when the children do not accept earphones. Although speech stimuli often are more relevant for the child than tonal stimuli, it is also important to obtain tonal threshold information for a "complete diagnostic picture." When testing within the sound field, standing waves may arise with use of pure-tone stimuli which may interfere with stimulus calibration and accurate hearing measurement. Frequency modulated (FM) and/or pulsed signals of various frequencies, often 500 Hz to 4000 Hz, lead to more accurate measurement and may be presented when implementing BOA techniques. Although sound field measurements yield valuable information, the child should be closely followed and individual-ear information attained as soon as diagnostically possible.

Because children of this age are unable to lateralize with a head turn or offer more overt behavioral responses, the audiologist searches for very subtle behavioral changes. These may include grimacing, increased or decreased pacifier sucking, crying, a cessation of activity, or eye shifting. The experienced clinician seeks a time-locked response on the part of the child. That is, the child's subtle behavioral response should occur in proper temporal sequence following the stimulus presentation, as opposed to appearing too quickly or too delayed. Audiology literature has described a "listening attitude," although its identification is subjective and may not withstand the tests of evidence-based practice time. Audiologists who have used BOA techniques within pediatric settings have welcomed the advent of more objective and interpretable measures: electrophysiology and more reliable behavioral techniques. Clinicians may recall roller coasterlike testing sessions with BOA: instances of elation when increased sucking was noted in response to a stimulus, followed by doubt when no response was seen to the same stimulus, and followed again by increased sucking behavior when no stimulus was presented. When testing children, two examiners are often necessary. One audiologist typically is situated outside of the sound suite in order to manipulate controls of the audiometer and present the calibrated test stimuli. The other audiologist is situated inside the booth so that he or she may, in the case of BOA, help keep the infant and parent in the proper position for testing. The two audiologists must be in continual communication with one another, to determine progression of test protocols and to interpret responses. One of the most important roles of the second examiner, in close proximity to the child, is to help interpret the child's responses. Parental participation may also play an integral role in comforting the child and in response interpretation. Because the parent is most familiar with the child and his behaviors, the parent may be the best determinant of subtle behavioral changes. The parent must be extensively counseled regarding withholding his or her own responses to stimuli presented and inadvertent provision of cues to the child. As both pure-tone and speech stimuli may be presented via the sound field, the parent is able to hear them and may unintentionally react, particularly if they are sufficiently intense. In addition, parents may intentionally repeat the stimuli or provide additional clues to the pediatric patient, in an attempt to elicit response.

Visual Reinforcement Audiometry (VRA)

The pediatric audiologist, with extensive auditory development knowledge, rejoices when a lateralization to sound to either the right or left develops at the approximate developmental age of six months. At this magical milestone, Visual Reinforcement Audiometry (VRA) may be implemented behaviorally and this technique may result in well-constructed audiograms. The infant is seated on a parental or other lap, at a calibrated location within the sound suite. Presentation of stimuli is typically through loudspeaker at first, although the importance of obtaining individual ear information cannot be overestimated. Deviations may be made from the audiologist's conventional protocol, with speech audiometry often conducted first. Test protocols with any patient may vary from audiologist to audiologist, with some routinely performing pure-tone audiometry first and others routinely beginning the testing session with speech audiometry. Speech stimuli are often more meaningful than pure-tone stimuli to a small child, with the child's name and other familiar words more likely to yield successful results.

One examiner is seated within the booth, typically in front of the child to keep the head at midline by distracting him with a bag of interesting toys. A conditioning process takes place whereby the examiner at the audiometer presents monitored live-voice speech stimuli through the microphone at a suprathreshold intensity level. On hearing, the examiner inside the booth immediately helps the child lateralize toward the appropriate speaker, followed by reinforcing the child with a lighted, animated toy. After several conditioning trials, the clinician extinguishes the helping behavior, hoping a conditioned bond has been established and that the child may perform the lateralization task on his own. In settings where two audiologists are not present, a technician may be present inside the sound suite to assist and/or the parent may also provide valuable support. Following conditioning, the examiner quickly descends in intensity to ascertain threshold with the child receiving no further help from the other clinician in eliciting the response. The audiologists make certain that the child is conditioned before descending in intensity and initiating the threshold-obtaining procedure.

Although the examiners utilize a modified Hughson-Westlake procedure for obtaining threshold, they must adapt by descending and bracketing threshold in a time-efficient manner. Also, they may accept fewer responses than the targeted 50% criterion used with adult patients and older children, prior to progressing along to the subsequent test stimulus. The time-efficiency and acceptance of fewer responses relate to limited attention span of the child and the need to progress efficiently, obtaining as much valid diagnostic information as possible. Figure 7–1 shows a small child being tested via VRA techniques.

Once a Speech Awareness Threshold (SAT) is obtained within the sound field, the audiologist progresses toward obtaining thresholds with warble tone stimuli. With such stimuli, the frequency modulates about the center frequency. In deviating from the traditional pure-tone protocol, audiologists often feel fortunate to obtain pediatric thresholds from 500 to 4000 Hz, as opposed to the entire frequency range. Audiologic information at other test frequencies is certainly important, if the child's attention span allows it to be obtained. Furthermore, the audiologist may change the order of frequencies

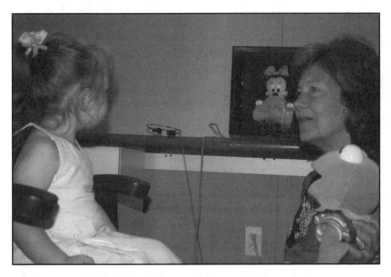

Figure 7–1. Young child being tested via visual reinforcement audiometry (VRA).

tested, testing a high frequency after testing 1 kHz and then "filling in the frequency gaps" as the child's attention span allows. When testing within the sound field, one must recall that results may reflect performance of a better ear and that it is important to obtain individual ear information as soon as possible. One may obtain sound field responses completely within normal limits, even in the presence of a profound unilateral hearing loss in one ear. The examiner must also recall the correct audiometric symbol to utilize, when recording sound field audiometric thresholds.

On establishing rapport and obtaining several sound field thresholds, the audiologist may attempt earphone or insert receiver placement for obtaining individual ear information. Many audiologists are successful with use of very small insert earphones with children, whereas others prefer supra-aural earphones that may require top-of-the-head cushion placement for proper fit. Some small children do not seem to realize that a head turn is still possible when wearing earphones; they may require demonstration that they may still exhibit a head turn with earphones in place in alliance with VRA techniques. If individual ear SATs are obtained, the audiologist may wish to then obtain higher frequency thresholds (2 kHz, 4 kHz) after transitioning to tonal testing. Just as the clinician may wish to alter test frequency progression to obtain high, mid, and low frequency information, he may wish to switch ears after obtaining each threshold. If a child chooses to end the session after obtaining four thresholds because of limited attention span, it is better to have recorded two for each ear instead of four for one ear and none for the other.

With regard to VRA, the examiner outside the booth who manipulates audiometer controls often also controls the animated toys. Great clinical insight is necessary to gain speed without forfeiting accuracy and to efficiently interpret pediatric responses. Responses should be appropriately time-locked according to stimulus presentation, with immediate reinforcement provided. False-positive responses should not be rewarded. The distracting toys, meant to keep the head at midline, should not be so interesting that the child prefers playing with them over lateralizing to the lighted toy. Challenges in bringing the head back to midline may occur with those children who find the lighted toy so fascinating that they do not wish to avert gaze. Children may require reconditioning during the testing session and may habituate to the lighted toy, finding it to no longer be novel or interesting. When this occurs, the audiologist may alter animation-light combinations, may implement a novel auditory stimulus, may recondition, or may introduce a new visual reinforcement toy. Although VRA techniques may be used through approximately the developmental age of two years, attending may be challenging for children at the upward end of this age range. As with any technique and especially with those where sound field stimuli are presented, parents must be instructed not to respond to stimuli and thereby interfere with the testing session. Occasionally, the audiologist encounters children who may not be conditioned to tasks required and for whom behavioral results may not be obtained. Referral for electrophysiologic measures is in order in these cases, especially after several attempts at behavioral testing, so that the identification process is not delayed.

Conditioned Play Audiometry (CPA)

Once a child reaches preschool age (approximate developmental age of 3–5 years old), he or she may be tested via Conditioned Play Audiometry (CPA). A child of this age will usually wear earphones, although the clinician may wish to condition the child within the sound field first. The child may be more apt to accept earphones if tried on a parent first, if described as Mickey Mouse™ ears, or if compared to those that airplane pilots wear. Two examiners are often needed, with one inside the booth with the child and one manipulating audiometer controls, although a solo audiologist may test from inside the booth with a portable audiometer. With a single-examiner method, manipulation of audiometer controls including stimulus presentation must be outside the child's line of sight. The premise behind CPA is to create an enjoyable game, with endless possibilities existing for positive response to test stimuli: dropping a block into a box on hearing the stimulus, placing a ring on a peg, building a tower one floor at a time, constructing a chain one link at a time, and many others. Speech audiometry may be performed first, as a more interesting stimulus, and the child is once again conditioned at a suprathreshold level to tasks required. On hearing the speech stimulus, often a phrase such as "put it in" expressed via monitored live voice, the child receives examiner assistance in performing the necessary play-based task. After much reinforcement and several conditioning trials, the audiologist working with the child makes certain that the child performs the task without assistance. This is the point where a conditioned bond is well established and the threshold-obtaining procedure may begin. A modified Hughson-Westlake procedure may be used, with clinicians working efficiently to descend in intensity toward threshold and possibly to accept fewer positive responses to achieve the necessary 50% criterion.

The audiologist inside the sound suite wears an ear monitor to ascertain when stimuli are being presented and the two audiologists must communicate with one another regarding pacing and child response patterns. The audiologist outside the sound suite must make certain that the response is overt enough to observe and responses must be time-locked with regard to the stimulus. Both clinicians are expertly educated to also observe and interpret behavioral responses. Figure 7-2 demonstrates a testing session where CPA techniques are utilized.

Some children may not be conditioned to tasks required, even after numerous trials; in this case, the audiologist may attempt to evaluate utilizing another technique geared toward developmentally less advanced patients or may implement electrophysiologic techniques. Some children may require reconditioning throughout the testing session or may require a game change when attention span wanes.

Pure-tone testing is accomplished after obtaining of SATs, or Speech Recognition Thresholds (SRTs) if the child is capable of repeating spondee words or pointing to pictures. Speech and pure-tone thresholds provide complementary information and should be in good agreement with each other to ensure reliability of results. Pediatric audiologists are aware that less clinical time and effort are required to repeat speech audiometry measures, if agreement is poor, than to repeat the pure-tone audiogram. As with VRA, the audiologist feels fortunate when pure-tone thresholds from 500 to 4000 Hz are obtained and thereby may deviate from conventional methods of testing the entire frequency range. Certainly, thresholds at 250 and

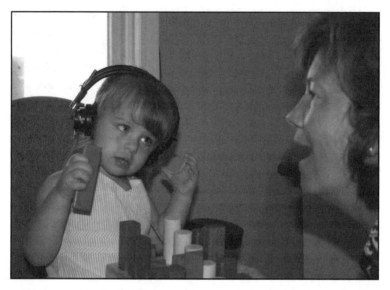

Figure 7–2. Young child being tested via conditioned play audiometry (CPA).

8000 Hz are important to measure when the child's attention span allows. The examiner may not proceed through the traditional frequency range in sequence, but may obtain thresholds within the middle and higher frequency ranges before "filling in the gaps" with additional test frequencies. Similarly, the clinician may alternate back and forth between ears so that audiologic information is obtained for both ears, in the event of child fatigue. Supra-aural earphones and/or insert receivers may be utilized with pediatric patients for AC testing. With older preschool-aged patients, the audiologist may also enhance the diagnostic battery by adding BC testing, masking if necessary, and assessment of word recognition abilities. Typically, the child's attention span allows both AC and BC testing and children adapt well to BC vibrator placement. The child also may be able either to point to pictures or to repeat words for word recognition testing. With regard to masking tasks, many children of this age are able to disregard the masking noise, while responding to the tonal or speech stimuli. When the child does not adapt to tasks required for masking, other components of the test battery as described in Chapter 6 provide valuable information regarding hearing status and characteristics. A child usually is able to perform conventional techniques during pure-tone audiometry by the time he reaches the developmental age of four to five years of age. That is, children of this age will readily raise a hand or push a button every time a tone is heard.

Immittance Audiometry

Although not a traditional pure-tone test, a pediatric audiology section would not be complete without a brief summary of immittance audiometry. Pure-tone signals play a major role in the two primary components of the immittance test battery: tympanometry and acoustic reflex testing. With tympanometry, the audiologist measures mobility of the middle ear system in response to air pressure change and also in response to a pure-tone that is delivered into the ear canal. Acoustic reflex testing measures function of the ipsilateral and contralateral acoustic reflex arcs by the probe's detection of compliance changes in response to high-intensity stimuli. Although immittance audiometry is beyond the scope of this text, it should be noted that high-intensity pure-tone stimuli from 500 to 4000 Hz are delivered via either probe or earphone in attempt to elicit the ipsilateral or contralateral Acoustic Reflex Threshold (ART). Immittance audiometry helps to supplement pure-tone audiometry by serving as one of the first objective measures within the audiologic test battery. Figure 7–3 demonstrates immittance audiometry being performed with a small child.

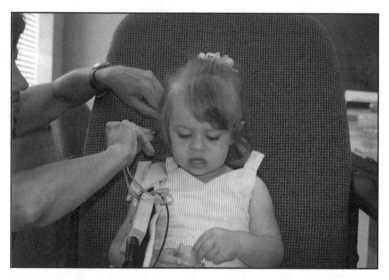

Figure 7–3. Performance of immittance audiometry with a small child.

TUNING FORK TESTS

Pure tones rarely occur within everyday listening situations, with most common sources being tuning forks and pure-tone audiometric signals. Tuning fork tests traditionally have been used for screening purposes by medical personnel, including audiologists, and/or for gaining additional diagnostic information regarding hearing status. They may assist to complement results obtained on the audiogram and to assist in interpretation, as well as the diagnostic process. Although they may not determine magnitude of hearing loss, they may indicate type: conductive versus sensorineural. Tuning forks represent various frequencies at octave intervals and vibrate following striking, with signal amplitude directly related to force. Tuning fork tests may especially provide clinical insights with challenging-to-test populations and may help confirm results of other diagnostic measures. Although usually termed "tuning fork tests," some may also be performed with the bone conduction oscillator of the audiometer. As with many procedures, they should not be used in isolation or take the place of pure-tone audiometry. Four major tuning fork tests are briefly described (Johnson, 1970; Martin & Clark, 2009).

The Bing test is based on the occlusion effect, a phenomenon where the listener perceives bone conducted stimuli as being louder, as a result of closing off the ear canal opening. The examiner strikes the tuning fork, holds it next to the mastoid bone behind the pinna, and alternately closes/opens the ear canal with a finger. A positive Bing finding is indicated if the occlusion effect is observed and the tone is perceived as louder on closing of the ear canal. Patients with an existing conductive pathology will experience a negative Bing finding, where the tone is not perceived as louder on occlusion effect, because the disorder is already resulting in such occlusion. The reader is referred to discussions of air and bone conducted stimuli and types of hearing loss that appear in Chapters 4 and 5.

The Rinne test involves striking of the tuning fork and alternately placing it on the mastoid for bone conduction hearing and at the ear canal opening for air conduction hearing. A positive Rinne finding occurs when the listener perceives that the tone is louder via air conduction than via bone conduction, as the former mode of hearing is more efficient. This finding may be present with normal hearing or with a patient demonstrating a sensorineural hearing loss. A negative Rinne finding occurs when the bone conducted stimulus appears to be louder than the air conducted stimulus and this may occur with a patient exhibiting a conductive hearing loss. As with many forms of audiologic testing, the clinician must be aware of nontest ear participation and take this into account during interpretation. A detailed discussion of such crossing over to the nontest ear appears in the clinical masking section in Chapter 6.

The Schwabach test involves placing the vibrating tuning fork on the mastoid of the patient and on that of the examiner, with an underlying assumption that the examiner displays normal hearing sensitivity. Quantification occurs by determining a difference in seconds between the tone no longer being heard by the patient and the tone no longer being heard by the clinician. A prolonged Schwabach finding occurs when the patient hears the tone for a longer duration than the examiner. In this case, a conductive loss is suspected. If the patient hears the tone for a shorter period of time than the clinician, a sensorineural hearing loss is suspected. Measurement is difficult, in that seconds must be counted and levels of significant difference determined.

The Weber test, modified for use with modern technology, is a test of lateralization where the patient must report if the tone is heard at midline, the right side, the left side, or in both ears. BC oscillator or tuning fork placement is often in the center of the forehead and patients are asked in which ear the stimulus appears louder. Normal listeners or those with symmetric (with regard to degree and type) hearing losses often report hearing the tone at midline. Patients with a unilateral sensorineural hearing loss often will hear the tone in the better ear, whereas patients with a unilateral conductive loss will hear the tone in the poorer ear. Various other patterns may exist and the audiologist must bear in mind that these results are subjective, exercising caution with instructions to avoid "leading" the patient toward anticipated results. Finally, the clinician must maintain a perspective of utilizing such findings in conjunction with all other important aspects of comprehensive, diagnostic audiologic techniques.

NONORGANIC HEARING LOSS

Occasionally, the audiologist tests a patient who may be voluntarily or involuntarily feigning a hearing impairment. This may be for a variety of reasons, including financial gain, the seeking of attention, psychological disorder, or others. This type of hearing impairment is referred to as "functional" or "nonorganic." The referral source may provide clues to the audiologist that the patient may demonstrate a functional hearing loss, as may information obtained during the case history interview. Valuable information also may be provided by observing unusual patient behaviors during the interview such as exaggerated straining to hear, displaying greater communication difficulty than in the waiting room, saying "yes" to every symptom that the audiologist brings forth, repeatedly referring to himself as "deaf," making excuses in advance for inconsistent test results, and asking about current compensation packages.

During the comprehensive audiologic evaluation, the audiologist may deviate from standard protocol with a functional hearing loss patient. The audiologist may perform speech audiometry prior to pure-tone testing and will seek agreement between speech and pure-tone thresholds. Lack of agreement may lend credence to presence of a nonorganic component; speech audiometry results may be better than pure-tone thresholds and may be a truer reflection of actual hearing sensitivity. A patient who is exaggerating a hearing loss may realize he or she should do so with tonal stimuli but not with speech stimuli. When performing pure-tone testing, an ascending threshold-obtaining procedure may be implemented where stimulus intensity begins at a subthreshold level. With this method, the patient may not "loudness match" as readily as he or she may with a descending procedure. Instead of button-pushing or hand-raising tasks, some audiologists have chosen to utilize a "yes" or "no" response. One may imagine a clinician's satisfaction when a patient consistently denies hearing a tone, each time one is presented. Unusual behaviors also may be observed during the actual testing session, such as straining to hear, attempting to hold the earphone closer to the ear, repeating only half of a two-syllable spondee word, displaying extremely delayed responses, exhibiting inconsistencies, demonstrating no crossing over to the nontest ear when this should be occurring, and many others. Responses to either tonal or speech stimuli may be very inconsistent. Often, counseling and reinstruction of the patient on the part of the audiologist will yield more accurate results on retest. At other times, special tests may be in order. Objective tests, such as Auditory Brainstem Response (ABR), Otoacoustic Emissions (OAEs), and Acoustic Reflexes may be helpful in elucidating nonorganic hearing loss.

The Stenger test is a special test that may utilize either speech or pure-tone stimuli for helping to determine presence of functional hearing loss. This test is based on the Stenger phenomenon where identical tones are presented to the two ears simultaneously. When this occurs, the listener only perceives the louder as opposed to the two individual stimuli. The Stenger test may be performed in special cases of exaggerating a unilateral hearing impairment where the admitted threshold in the "poorer ear" is 20 dB or more poorer than the admitted threshold in the "better ear." Although there are many testing variations, a first step is to present a tonal stimulus to the better ear at +10 dB SL (re: pure-tone threshold), following instructions to indicate when a tone is heard. The examiner presents instructions in a simplified manner, omitting delineation of each step and the theory on which the test is based, so as not to interfere with test efficiency or outcome. The audiologist anticipates a positive response following the first step. The second step involves presenting a tone of the same frequency to the poorer ear at −10 dB SL (re: pure-tone threshold). Because this level is 10 dB below the admitted threshold, the audiologist anticipates no response. The third and final step involves presenting both stimuli to the two ears at the intensity levels already described. If the admitted threshold in the poorer ear is not accurate, the patient will only hear the tone in this ear and will not be aware of the tone presented in the better ear. He or she will not respond, just as in step two, and this is termed a positive Stenger finding. On the other hand, the admitted threshold in the poorer ear may be a true threshold. If this is the case, the patient will not hear the tone presented in the poorer ear and will respond to the tone presented in the better ear. A positive response therefore yields a negative Stenger result and the patient is thought to demonstrate a true hearing impairment.

Pure-tone stimuli applications in audiology are wide and varied, including those described with functional hearing loss patients. The audiologist may also make clinical judgments regarding true hearing status following conversation at normal intensity levels through the audiometer's microphone or word recognition testing at very soft intensity levels. The audiologist should exercise caution with report writing and only report factual results, as opposed to impressions that may not be based on objective evidence obtained during the testing session. Case documentation should always be extensive and thorough.

ULTRAHIGH-FREQUENCY AUDIOMETRY

The audiologist may occasionally perform pure-tone audiometry at frequencies higher than 8 kHz, through use of a high-frequency audiometer. Clinical implications include identifying effects of oto-toxic agents and disorders that primarily affect the basal end of the cochlea, responsible for perception of higher frequency information. Early detection of changes in the extended high-frequency region and prior to the occurrence of changes in conventional audiometric frequencies may have important ramifications toward case management. ANSI S3.6 (2004) defines such extended high-frequency audiometer utility as especially useful with pure-tone threshold measurement from 8 kHz to 16 kHz. Although equipment varies, these special audiometers may incorporate test frequencies up to 18 or 20 kHz. Figure 7–4 shows a high-frequency audiometer, illustrating the frequency dial, intensity dial, and special earphones that must be utilized with such testing. Annex C of *ANSI S3.6 (2004) Specifications for Audiometers* delineates specific requirements for calibration of

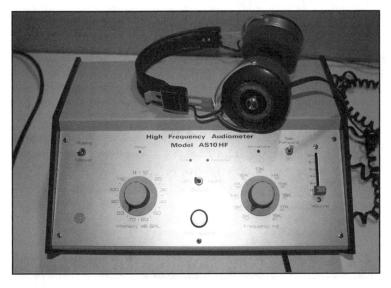

Figure 7–4. Extended frequency audiometer showing primary controls and circumaural earphones.

circumaural earphones that are used with extended high frequency testing. The clinician must be aware of special calibration issues that may be encountered with this equipment and emission of such high-frequency signals (Stelmachowicz, Gorga, & Cullen, 1982; Stelmachowicz, Beauchaine, Kalberer, Larger, & Jesteadt, 1988).

The primary clinical application of such testing is with patients who are exposed to ototoxic agents and who are undergoing resultant audiologic monitoring programs. This is because hearing changes occur in the upper spectrum of the frequency range prior to occurring in the more traditional speech frequencies. Ototoxicity may be acquired, such as when a patient is prescribed medications or is exposed to environmental toxins that may result in cochlear damage. There is also a form of congenital ototoxicity, whereby a mother passes effects of ototoxic agents to her unborn child. Examples of ototoxic medications are many and the audiologist must remain current with regard to the list of medications and their effects. Some medications may be more cochleotoxic and may result in detrimental effects on hearing, whereas others affect vestibular function due to vestibulotoxic effects. Examples of ototoxic medications include the family of strong aminoglycoside antibiotics, loop diuretics, strong doses of aspirin, antimalarial drugs including quinine, some chemotherapies, and others. In addition to gaining pharmacology knowledge related to ototoxic medications, it is also the audiologist's responsibility to work as a team with physicians and other medical personnel who help manage these patients. As the audiologist monitors and notes effects on hearing, the audiologist communicates to other medical personnel and the treatment course may possibly be altered.

Prior to medication administration, it is important to obtain baseline pure-tone audiometry information whenever possible. The audiologist is instrumental in development of a regular monitoring program. This monitoring protocol is individualized and dependent on many factors: patient, medication, dosage, medical team preferences, and others. ASHA (2005) recommends that threshold assessment at the following traditional test frequencies be included with monitoring programs: 500 Hz, 1 kHz, 2 kHz, 3 kHz, 4 kHz, 6 kHz, 8 kHz, and at other test frequencies as appropriate. The ototoxic monitoring protocol, of course, would also include frequencies within the extended range. Often, serial audiogram forms are utilized whereby the audiologist numerically records threshold as a function of frequency and day/time of evaluation, thereby facilitating comparison of threshold over time. This is in contrast to more standard audiogram forms and recording with utilization of traditional audiometric symbols. The audiologist also may perform baseline OAEs and perform regular OAE monitoring of hair cell function.

There are a number of clinical insights that the audiologist must bear in mind when testing this very special population. As one listens to the ultrahigh-frequency stimuli, one notes that they may lose their tonal quality and that the stimulus at times sounds more noiselike. Extended range audiometers may be calibrated to dB SPL, as opposed to dB HL. Interpretation with caution must be exercised as the clinician considers nonlinearity properties of the ear and the sound pressure level that must be exerted before threshold is attained at the high frequencies. Adult patients especially may demonstrate no response to stimuli at the limits of the high-frequency audiometer equipment, even during the baseline phase, causing subsequent monitoring to be an impossible task.

It is important to remember that each patient's case must be individually managed, in that there is individual susceptibility to ototoxic agents. Harmful effects of medication may be related to such entities as daily dosage, cumulative dosage, duration of treatment, renal function, synergistic effects with noise and other agents, and a variety of other factors. Often, such medications are prescribed because there is a life-threatening illness. In such cases, hearing and/or vestibular function may be sacrificed in an attempt to save the patient's life. High-frequency audiometry patients often are inpatients who are quite ill and may not adapt readily to conventional techniques required for pure-tone audiometry. The serious medical condition may be such that assessment and management of hearing loss may not be a medical priority of the patient or family. In addition to skill and knowledge required for effective assessment, the audiologist must also exercise a high level of competence and empathy. The audiologist must work diplomatically as a team member with other medical personnel and must compassionately work with critically ill patients. The test environment may be altered, in that many patients are seen at bedside and may be housed within an intensive care unit. Fortunately, high-frequency thresholds are quite valid as the audiometer is accompanied by circumaural earphones and there is a stimulus release from masking amidst the primarily lower frequency noise levels. In addition, baseline and monitoring thresholds typically are obtained within a constant environment and this allows comparisons to readily be made. When threshold changes are noted during the monitoring process, the physician is notified and it may be possible to change medications and/or dosages.

In 1994, the American Speech-Language-Hearing Association published guidelines for patients receiving ototoxic medications. They include:

1. Establishing criteria for toxicity identification
2. Identifying at-risk patients within a timely manner
3. Counseling regarding effects, prior to beginning of treatment
4. Valid baseline measures performed preferably before treatment (or shortly thereafter)
5. Monitoring at intervals with documentation of hearing impairment and its progression
6. Follow-up post-treatment evaluation to determine any detrimental effects and plan management strategies.

CONCLUSIONS

Pure-tone audiometry has great clinical utility with challenging-to-test and other unique populations. Conventional techniques, such as hand-raising and button-pushing, may be altered when the patient is unable to adapt to tasks required. The development of electro-physiologic techniques was a major milestone within the field, particularly with regard to early identification of hearing loss with young children who could not yet be evaluated behaviorally. Auditory Brainstem Response (ABR) testing and Otoacoustic Emissions (OAEs) have gained extraordinary clinical utility with helping to estimate hearing threshold. Both implement pure-tones in the form of very brief tone-bursts for elicitation of desired waveform responses.

By the time a child reaches the approximate developmental age of six months, he or she may be efficiently tested via behavioral testing techniques. Both Visual Reinforcement Audiometry (VRA) and Conditioned Play Audiometry (CPA) involve delivery of either pure-tone or warble-tone stimuli, dependent on the transducer. It is important for the audiologist to attempt threshold measures for both pure-tone and speech stimuli, as these results serve to complement one another. Many young children may be evaluated via conventional techniques by the age of 4 to 5 years and also may readily adapt to tasks required for masking procedures.

The audiologist may also alter the more standard pure-tone testing protocol, depending on needs of individual patients. Expert clinical insights are important in these cases, as the audiologist determines best practice protocols for each individualized clinical situation. There may be instances when the audiologist performs speech audiometry before pure-tone testing or performs an ascending technique, in lieu of the modified Hughson-Westlake procedure. For example, with geriatric or cognitively disabled clients, the clinician may perform speech audiometry first and may streamline conventional pure-tone protocols. The audiologist also may implement various tuning fork tests to supplement information attained via other diagnostic measures. These measures may be especially helpful in determining type of hearing impairment.

With patients suspected of demonstrating functional hearing loss, the audiologist may perform speech audiometry prior to pure-tone testing and may choose an ascending method for all threshold determinations. With functional hearing loss patients, the audiologist also may choose to utilize more objective measures that incorporate pure-tone stimuli. Examples of these tests are the Acoustic Reflex Threshold (ART) and the Auditory Brainstem Response (ABR). Additional special tests are available, such as the Stenger test, that use pure-tone stimuli and that help determine presence of functional hearing loss.

Audiologists play a major role in management of patients who are receiving medications and other substances that may be ototoxic. The clinician must be well versed on ototoxic medications and other agents and must serve as an important member of the hearing health care team. With regard to evaluation, a baseline evaluation prior to administration is critical and often involves extended high-frequency audiometry via specialized equipment. In addition to pure-tone audiometry that is performed at traditional audiometric frequencies, the audiologist adds pure-tone audiometry from 8 kHz through 16 to 18 kHz to the diagnostic battery. Detrimental effects on hearing sensitivity may be seen in this frequency region prior to the lower frequency region. It is the audiologist's role to detect and articulate these changes. It is clear that pure-tone audiometry provides the foundation for comprehensive diagnostic evaluation and serves as a springboard for technique adaptation and for additional complex and sophisticated diagnostic measures.

REFERENCES

American National Standards Institute. (2004). *Specifications for audiometers (S3.6-2004)*. New York: Acoustical Society of America.

American Speech-Language-Hearing Association. (1994). Guidelines for audiologic management of individuals receiving cochleotoxic drug therapy. *Asha, 36*, 11-19.

American Speech-Language-Hearing Association. (2005). *Guidelines for manual pure-tone threshold audiometry*. Rockville, MD: Author.

Goldstein, R., & Aldrich, W. M. (1999). *Evoked potential audiometry: Fundamentals and applications*. Boston: Allyn & Bacon.

Johnson, E. W. (1970). Tuning forks to audiometers and back again. *Laryngoscope, 80*, 49-68.

Kemp, D. T. (1979). Evidence of mechanical nonlinearity and frequency selective wave amplification in the cochlea. *Archives of Oto-Rhino-Laryngology, 221*, 37-45.

Martin, F. N., & Clark, J. G. (2009). *Introduction to audiology* (10th ed.). Boston: Pearson.

Stelmachowicz, P. G., Beauchaine, K. A., Kalberer, A., Langer, T., & Jesteadt, W. (1988). The reliability of auditory thresholds in the 8- to 20-kHz range using a prototype audiometer. *Journal of the Acoustical Society of America, 83,* 1528–1535.

Stelmachowicz, P. G., Gorga, M. P., & Cullen, J. K. (1982). A calibration procedure for the assessment of thresholds above 8000 Hz. *Journal of Speech and Hearing Research, 25,* 618–623.

8 Identification Audiometry: Hearing Screening

The audiologist must differentiate between screening and evaluation with regard to pure-tone audiometry and many other areas of practice. A screening is a quick and efficient measure, designed for implementation with large groups, to determine need for a thorough evaluation. It may be performed by personnel outside the audiology profession, under an audiologist's supervision; for example, the speech-language pathologist may perform a hearing screening prior to a speech and language evaluation to determine possible effects of hearing status on a speech and/or language disorder. In 1997, the American Speech-Language-Hearing Association (ASHA) published *Guidelines for Audiometric Screening*, an in-depth set of recommendations for conducting hearing screening across the life span. The Joint Committee on Infant Hearing published a revised Position Statement in 2007 outlining extensive guidelines related to hearing screening and early intervention.

Many important principles must be considered in development of a screening program. There must be measurable definition of the disorder and effective treatments must be available. Screening protocols in general are highly effective with disease courses that are altered by early identification and intervention, such as exist within the audiology profession. Screening tools must be time-efficient, cost-effective, sensitive, and specific. Sensitivity refers to probability of obtaining positive test results with those patients actually displaying a disorder, whereas specificity refers to probability of obtaining negative test results with those who do not display the disorder.

This chapter focuses on pure-tone hearing screening with older children and adults, as the reader is referred to another textbook in this series that focuses on infant hearing screening. Although emphasizing infant hearing, many principles outlined in the 2007 Joint Committee Position Statement may be applied to patient evaluation and treatment across the life span. Patients who undergo hearing screening should receive appropriate follow-up for confirmation of hearing loss within a timely manner. In addition to establishing efficient initial screening protocols, the audiologist must establish thorough protocols for rescreening and follow-up diagnostic services. When a patient does not pass a hearing screening, he or she should be scheduled for a comprehensive audiologic evaluation with an audiologist. Remediation services should also be initiated immediately following diagnosis of hearing impairment, preferably with a single point of entry into the intervention system. Family-centered, informed choices should be provided to the patient through a team approach that explicitly outlines all treatment options and extensive counseling. High-quality technology should optimally be available to all patients, as related to audiologic evaluation and (re)habilitative measures. Hearing impairment of all patients should be closely monitored within his or her medical home, interfacing when possible with electronic health records for optimal data entry and management.

An expanded definition of hearing loss, outlined in the Joint Committee Position Paper (2007), also applies across the life span and includes permanent bilateral sensorineural, unilateral sensorineural, permanent conductive, and neural hearing losses. The ASHA Guidelines (1997) thoroughly address the life span, incorporating five major sections for pediatric screening: middle ear disorders, infants from 0 to 6 months of age, infants from 7 months through two years of age, preschool populations from three to five years of age, and school-aged populations. The final section relates to adult populations, incorporating recommended screening protocols to denote impairment, disability, and disorder.

It is important that all test procedures be thoroughly explained to the patient or to the guardian of a minor patient and that the party willingly participates. Infection control must be utilized, equipment must be properly calibrated, and daily listening checks must be rigorously performed prior to screening. As with any evaluative procedure, accurate documentation and patient record-keeping must be employed. An audiologist should design and manage the screening program, with regular evaluation of program effectiveness. Although audiologists primarily engage in thorough diagnostic work, there are clinical occasions when the audiologist performs and/or supervises hearing screenings.

Prior to performing the hearing screening, it is recommended that the examiner obtain brief case history information and perform otoscopy. Scope of practice is an important consideration with various aspects of screening protocols: some aspects may only be performed by an audiologist whereas others may be performed by other disciplines under an audiologist's supervision.

SCREENING FOR OUTER AND MIDDLE EAR DISORDERS

The importance of combining immittance screening with pure-tone screening is readily apparent, particularly with younger children. The immittance screening likely will identify a child with otitis media (or other middle ear disorder) who may have passed a pure-tone screening and who may consequently demonstrate speech, language, and/or academic difficulty due to a mild hearing impairment. Children who are at risk especially should be screened, with such risk factors including areas such as bottle feeding, first bout of otitis media with effusion prior to six months of age, enrollment in daycare, exposure to secondhand smoke, craniofacial anomalies, and ethnic populations with higher incidence. Pure-tone stimuli are utilized as an important component during performance of tympanometry and acoustic reflex testing. Professionals who perform immittance screenings devise criteria for rescreening and/or medical referral. Screening procedures must be efficient and accurate, documentation must be thorough, and appropriate follow-up measures must be undertaken.

SCREENING OF INFANTS FROM BIRTH TO SIX MONTHS

The Joint Committee on Infant Hearing advocated the goal in 1994 to detect infants with hearing impairment as soon as possible, so that early intervention may begin. Within 15 years, most states had adopted universal hearing newborn screening and related follow-up programs. Although detailed discussion of infant hearing screening programs is beyond the scope of this textbook, there is relevance to pure-tone audiometry. As conventional techniques may not be utilized with this population, audiometric techniques have been adapted for use with such challenging populations. Specifically within the first six months of life, (electro)physiologic screening measures are recommended, performed by either an audiologist or support personnel under an audiologist's supervision.

Factors that place a child at risk for significant hearing impairment include: low Apgar scores, bacterial meningitis, congenital maternal infections, craniofacial anomalies, low birthweight, elevated bilirubin, administration of ototoxic medications, and others (ASHA, 1997). Many at-risk children may continue to be at risk for developing delayed-onset hearing impairment and should be closely followed at least every six months through the age of at least three years. Documentation of all results is imperative and special skill is required in counseling parents regarding results, particularly when a child does not pass the screening. It is important to make certain that the facility maintains family contact information and makes every possible effort to ensure that the patient returns for follow-up care.

SCREENING OF TODDLERS: 7 MONTHS THROUGH 2 YEARS

This is a challenging population to screen, although behavioral tests may be employed. Screening should primarily be performed by an audiologist, targeting those children who require follow-up care following a previous screening and/or those children who demonstrate risk factors previously listed. The key clinical process involves conditioning children to Visual Reinforcement Audiometric (VRA) techniques within the sound suite. As with threshold obtaining procedures, such screening procedures involve conditioning the child to tasks required at suprathreshold presentation levels. Upon hearing the stimulus, the child lateralizes toward the right or left and is visually reinforced with a lighted toy. Several examiners often are necessary while the child is seated on a parent lap, with one clinician manipulating audiometer controls (including the visual reinforcement) and another engaging the child. This second clinician is situated within the sound suite and distracts the child with interesting toys, while also keeping the head at midline. Upon a time-locked head turn response, the audiologist outside the booth reinforces the child with a lighted and/or animated toy. It is important to screen with pure-tone stimuli so that individual frequency information may be obtained. Supra-aural or insert earphones should be used according to child adaptation, so that individual ear information may be obtained. The audiologist may find it necessary to condition and begin screening the child in the sound field, prior to attempting earphone testing, in which case warble-tone stimuli are used.

Once the child is conditioned, the audiologist rapidly descends in intensity level to a stimulus presentation level that has been pre-determined to be the screening level. Instead of using the modified Hughson-Westlake method to ascertain exact threshold, stimuli are presented at a specific level and the child either responds or does not respond. With a screening procedure, pure-tone signals of specific frequencies are selected instead of presenting the entire audiometric frequency range as with a full evaluation. Frequencies recommended for screening with this population are 1 kHz, 2 kHz, and 4 kHz whereas the recommended presentation level is 30 dB HL. Screening procedures often do not include 500 Hz because ambient noise is also composed of low-frequency information and may mask the signal. Audiology clinics may devise their own screening forms that include a table similar to that shown in Figure 8–1. Additional information noted on the form may include identifying information, immittance screening results, brief summary of case history and/or otoscopic examination, and follow-up recommendations.

A "+" is recorded every time there is a positive response at screening level and a "–" is recorded every time the child does not respond. The child passes the screening if clinically reliable

	500 Hz	1 kHz	2 kHz	4 kHz
Right Ear				
Left Ear				

Presentation Level: _____ dB HL

+ denotes positive response   – denotes negative response

Pass _____   Refer _____

Follow-up Recommendations: _____

Figure 8–1. Example of form for recording hearing screening results.

responses are seen at the desired screening intensity level in each ear for each frequency. The child refers if no reliable response is seen at the screening level at any frequency in either ear. Too often the examiner descends in intensity prior to proper conditioning; it is critical to make certain the child is conditioned to tasks required prior to lowering presentation intensity level for the actual screening. Each positive response should be repeated for reliability purposes, rather than accepting only one positive response prior to sweeping through to the next frequency. Some precocious children within this age group may adapt to Conditioned Play Audiometry (CPA) techniques, as discussed in the subsequent section. Conversely, other children may not condition to tasks required for VRA due to developmental or other reasons and must be referred for ABR and/or OAE testing.

Certain procedures are not appropriate and these include usage of Behavioral Observation Audiometry, implementation of uncalibrated signals, and usage of broadband frequency stimuli such as speech signals. A speech threshold may certainly provide valuable information within confines of an evaluation, but should complement pure-tone findings and not serve as a substitute measure. Parents and guardians whose children refer on the screenings should be extensively counseled and follow-up procedures should be initiated. The screening audiologist should properly document all findings, provide counseling and educational materials, and schedule a follow-up appointment as soon as possible for rescreening or full evaluation in attempt to confirm presence of hearing impairment.

During counseling, the audiologist should bear in mind the purpose and limitations of a screening. Although a child who refers may be suspected of demonstrating a hearing impairment, this must be confirmed. A screening may indicate that a tonal stimulus was not heard at a specific level, but does not provide information regarding magnitude or type of hearing loss. If the child does not accept earphones and the screening is performed within the sound field, the audiologist is unable to explain individual ear information to parents and/or guardians. A screening level of 30 dB HL is recommended with this age group as they are typically less vigilant than older children and levels of detection often are elevated. Responses seen with young children may be "minimal response levels." When such a 30 dB HL criterion is utilized, there may be some instances where milder hearing losses may go undetected.

SCREENING OF PRESCHOOL-AGED CHILDREN

Screening of children within this age group is very commonly performed, either in large groups or as an integral part of a speech-language evaluation. Because many such screenings are performed outside a sound suite, the audiologist should make certain that the testing environment is as quiet as possible. Stories abound regarding audiologists who report to schools and preschools as part of a hearing screening team, only to be shown to a noisy gymnasium or boiler room. With this age group's high incidence of otitis media, it is also important to couple immittance screening with the pure-tone screening procedures. Personnel may include audiologists, speech-language pathologists, and support personnel under close supervision of an audiologist.

This group of children should be screened if risk factors are present, if there is a possibility of delayed-onset hearing loss, or if qualified professionals see additional need. Conditioned Play Audiometry (CPA) is the targeted technique in that most preschoolers are able to adapt to tasks required. As thoroughly outlined in Chapter 7, most children of this age will readily wear insert or supra-aural earphones for air conduction testing. The examiner brings to the session a wide array of toys for play audiometry, so that the child may be conditioned to place a ring on a peg, drop a block into a box, or perform a similar response on hearing the stimulus. In addition to securing an environment that is free of auditory distraction, the screening duo should also be free of visual distraction. As may be imagined, a row or line of classmates may be very distracting and interesting to a four-year-old. A common error is to fail to spend enough time on establishing a conditioned bond; the clinician should make certain he or she has engaged in enough conditioning trials to ascertain establishment of the conditioned bond. Once this bond is apparent, the audiologist may descend to the screening intensity level.

Recommended screening frequencies again are 1 kHz, 2 kHz, and 4 kHz. This is especially true because such screenings are frequently outside of sound booths and ambient noise interferes with tonal perception at 500 Hz. Should 500 Hz be incorporated into the screening protocol, one may anticipate overreferrals at that particular frequency. Because these children are older and better able to attend than those children described in the previous section, the recommended stimulus intensity level is 20 dB HL. Just as several conditioning trials are recommended prior to screening, several positive responses are required prior to moving along to the subsequent frequency. Responses may be recorded on a form similar to that shown in Figure 8–1.

It is not uncommon to note screening professionals obtaining AC thresholds while performing such a screening. This should be avoided, in view of the screening purpose and test environment. Rather, the method of choice is to sweep through recommended frequencies at the desired intensity level to determine presence or absence of a response. If a response is not present, the audiologist may wish to stop the test session for reinstruction. The author has found success in removing earphones, reinstructing the child to listen for a "very soft tone," presenting a stimulus at the suprathreshold conditioning level, and then descending to the screening intensity level. At times, there will be a positive response (which must be verified) after these measures whereas at other times there will continue to be no response.

The child passes the screening if reliable responses are seen following at least two out of three presentations, for each frequency and ear screened. The child should be referred for additional testing if two out of three positive responses are not noted or if the child is unable to adapt to CPA techniques. Although the child who does not accept earphones may be screened within the sound field, such equipment may not be available and one must also ultimately strive toward obtaining individual ear information. VRA may be utilized if the child does not respond to CPA behavioral techniques, although stimuli that lack frequency-specificity should be avoided.

When a child is referred, typical protocol is to schedule for a comprehensive audiologic evaluation to confirm presence of hearing loss as soon as possible. Within such a setting, teamwork involving many professional disciplines is necessary, as is providing in-depth educational materials to parents. As with any screening program, follow-up is imperative and the child may be referred for electrophysiologic measures if he or she cannot be tested behaviorally. Follow-through on the part of the audiologist and administrative personnel is critical, so that the child may receive the necessary evaluative and remediation measures.

SCREENING OF SCHOOL-AGED CHILDREN

Screening in the schools may be performed by an audiologist, speech-language pathologist or other support personnel under the supervision of a qualified audiologist. Immittance screening for identification of middle ear disorders should often accompany pure-tone screening, particularly in the kindergarten and early elementary grades. A portable audiometer is utilized for pure-tone screening, with the clinician seeking the quietest environment possible because a sound suite typically is not available. As with any other audiometric procedure, it is very important to ensure that the equipment is updated and in proper calibration. Recurrent threads continue to involve the obtaining of informed consent, especially as the parent or guardian may not be present during the testing session. The audiologist also must be aware of the need for universal precautions and infection control procedures, as well as the goal to screen large populations in an accurate and efficient manner.

This population should be screened on school enrollment, when the child is felt to be at risk, when there may be indications of a hearing loss reported, and when delayed-onset or progressive hearing loss is suspected. Among "at risk" factors may be admission into a special education program or recommendation to repeat a grade. Kindergarteners through third graders should be screened annually, according to ASHA Guidelines (1997). School-aged children should also undergo screening during the 7th and 11th grade years. With the advent of universal newborn hearing screening and early identification, many children have undergone hearing screening and evaluation prior to enrolling in school. This should not be assumed, however, and children who have never experienced screening should be targeted. Progressive or acquired hearing loss may also be present, such that school hearing screening is beneficial in identifying such cases, even when the child may have passed a hearing screening at birth.

Most children of school age may be evaluated via conventional, hand-raising techniques and most will accept earphones for ascertaining individual ear information. Children enrolled in earlier elementary grades may be tested via Conditioned Play Audiometric (CPA) techniques if attempts to condition to conventional techniques are unsuccessful. The standard screening frequencies of 1, 2, and 4 kHz are recommended with a screening presentation level of 20 dB HL. This screening level is sufficient if securing a quiet environment and because most children of this older age are able to listen for a softer stimulus that approaches threshold. Consistent with screening pass/refer criteria at other age levels, the child passes the screening when reliable responses are seen in each ear at each of the three test frequencies. On beginning the testing session and after providing instructions, the audiologist should present initial stimuli at intensity levels higher than 20 dB HL; once the student has adapted to the hand-raising task required, the audiologist may descend to the screening intensity level and proceed. A screening form similar to the one previously discussed may be utilized and the audiologist should ascertain presence of more than one reliable response before verifying that the screening was passed at that particular frequency. If no response to a stimulus is noted, it is helpful to reinstruct, reposition the earphones, and rescreen. The child should be referred to an audiologist for a thorough audiologic evaluation if he does not respond to a stimulus of any frequency presented to either ear or if he does not adapt to tasks required for screening.

Screening personnel should note that calibrated pure-tone stimuli are the stimuli of choice. Inappropriate procedures involve those that include use of speech stimuli as they do not provide frequency-specific information, noncalibrated stimuli, nontraditional or non-audiologic equipment, and group screening protocols. Similarly, electrophysiologic measures such as Otoacoustic Emissions (OAEs) and Auditory Brainstem Response (ABR) testing are not appropriate for hearing screening of school-aged children. The clinician should employ proper documentation and follow-up procedures, with the hearing loss identified as soon as possible (preferably within one month after screening and no later than three months postscreening). Screening personnel should bear in mind the need for immediate identification and intervention, in that even minimal hearing impairment may lead to significant academic, speech, and/or language difficulty. A team approach is imperative, with the audiologist counseling the student and contacting parents regarding audiologic results and recommendations. In-servicing of teachers and other school personnel regarding audiologic results and implementation of classroom remediation strategies is also imperative.

In addition to guidelines relevant to pure-tone screening, professionals working with school-aged children familiarize themselves with screening procedures for "disability." These procedures include identification of communication development delay, such as speech, language, academic, and behavioral disorders. The audiologist must recognize that many children demonstrate other disorders in addition to hearing impairment and the importance of working hand-in-hand with other disciplines toward team management.

SCREENING OF ADULTS

Audiologists, speech-language pathologists, and other support personnel may find themselves performing hearing screenings with adult clients. Examples might be with elderly populations who attend senior centers or who may reside in long-term health care facilities. Guidelines may be divided into three categories with all making valuable contributions toward the battery of evaluative measures: Disorders, Impairment, and Disability. Although all are important components, this section emphasizes pure-tone audiometry utilized when screening for hearing impairment.

Disorder

Screening for disorder involves identification of individuals who exhibit obvious physical anomalies of the ear and/or significant otologic history. This is often a first step in screening, in order to determine medical referral need as well as feasibility for proceeding with pure-tone screening. This aspect of screening involves a brief and face-to-face elicitation of pertinent case history information and visual examination of the outer ear structures via otoscopy. A patient passes the hearing screening for disorder if the inspection is negative for significant otologic findings whereas a medical referral is initiated if a positive and untreated symptom is identified.

Impairment

Pure-tone screening for impairment may be performed by a qualified audiologist, speech-language pathologist, or otherwise qualified support personnel under an audiologist's supervision. Individuals should be screened as requested and when history and environment may place them at risk, such as those exposed to work-related or recreational noise. Patients may be referred by a family member or may demonstrate a family history of hearing loss. ASHA (1997) also recommends that adults undergo hearing screening each decade through the age of 50 years and then every three years after the age of 50 years.

Conventional techniques typically are employed, with pure-tone stimuli delivered through insert or supra-aural earphones. Hearing screening is generally performed, in the quietest environment possible, at 1, 2, and 4 kHz with a presentation level of 25 dB HL. Initial stimuli should be presented at comfortable, suprathreshold levels as the patient adapts to tasks required and prior to the audiologist's descending to the designated screening level. The examiner should seek several positive responses at one frequency, as opposed to just one, before progressing to the subsequent screening step. When no response to a stimulus is seen, the audiologist should reinstruct, reposition the earphones, and rescreen. Screening forms should be similar to those discussed previously, including patient identification information and both ear-specific and frequency-specific information. As with all audiologic procedures, equipment should be in proper calibration and a daily listening check should be performed prior to initiating the screening procedure.

The hearing screening is passed when there are positive responses at all frequencies in both ears. The patient should be referred for a thorough audiologic evaluation when a negative response is seen at any frequency in either ear. The thorough audiologic evaluation may be optional if the patient passes the Disability Screening described in the next section or if the patient elects not to pursue further evaluation. Education and counseling regarding results are a very important component following a pure-tone screening. The audiologist must explicitly explain the purpose of a screening and that it does not allow the audiologist to determine magnitude or type of hearing loss. During the postscreening counseling session, the examiner explains that only a portion of the audiometric frequency range is tested. As opposed to finding thresholds, the screening determines whether hearing sensitivity is within or below normal limits. Furthermore, the audiologist explains that a thorough audiologic evaluation is the next step in helping to evaluate hearing impairment and determine remediation strategies: the need for medical referral, hearing aid evaluation, and other recommendations.

Disability

Occasionally, the audiologist works with a patient who either subjectively notes communication difficulty in the presence of a hearing screening for impairment "pass" or denies communication difficulty in the presence of a hearing screening "referral." A combination of subjective and objective data has become well utilized in various areas of audiologic practice. The audiologist who screens for disability may utilize a variety of short questionnaires that demonstrate documented internal and test-retest reliability. The questionnaire should be administered in a face-to-face format, intended to identify hearing disabilities that may adversely affect everyday listening environments: work-related, social, educational, and others. Examples of questionnaires that may be implemented are the Hearing Handicap Inventory for the Elderly–Screening Version (Ventry & Weinstein, 1983) and the Self-Assessment of Communication (Schow & Nerbonne, 1982). "Pass" versus "refer" score criteria are reported for both measures, for use as the screener develops his or her own screening protocols and criteria. Other measures exist in the literature and the audiologist must exercise caution to ensure that there are published data, demonstrated reliability, and established pass/refer guidelines.

Counseling, education, and follow-up are required with any high-quality adult hearing screening program. Screening personnel should refer for a thorough audiologic evaluation if the patient refers on either or both of the latter screening sections: screening for impairment and/or screening for disability.

CONCLUSIONS

Pure-tone audiometry plays an important role in identification through screening of patients who require thorough audiologic evaluation. Although screening may not commonly be performed in many settings and patients may be referred directly for thorough evaluation, the audiologist should be well versed in protocols, administration, interpretation and supervision of support personnel. This chapter has described screening practices across the life span, as well as personnel qualifications for various components. Pure-tone audiometry is directly implemented with many aspects of screening, including screening via Visual Reinforcement Audiometry, Conditioned Play Audiometry, and conventional techniques.

It is important to note major differences between administration of a thorough evaluation and a hearing screening. The purpose of a screening is to implement a quick and efficient procedure for identification of individuals requiring a more comprehensive workup. There are limitations in counseling one who "refers" on a screening, in that limited information is provided; however, effective counseling and follow-up are essential to ensure that targeted individuals receive required services. Although guidelines may be presented to the audiologist, he or she has acquired the vast knowledge and expertise to modify procedures and protocols, dependent on each individual circumstance, environment, and patient population.

REFERENCES

American Speech-Language-Hearing Association. (1997). *Guidelines for audiologic screening.* Rockville, MD: Author.

Joint Committee on Infant Hearing. (1994, December). Position statement. *Asha, 36,* 38–41.

Joint Committee on Infant Hearing. (2007). *Year 2007 position statement: Principles and guidelines for early hearing detection and intervention.* Available from www.asha.org/ policy

Schow, R. L., & Nerbonne, M. A. (1982). Communication Screening Profile: Use with elderly clients. *Ear and Hearing, 3,* 134–147.

Ventry, I., & Weinstein, B. (1983). Identification of elderly people with hearing problems. *Asha, 25,* 37–42.

9 *Sample Audiograms:*

Frequently Seen Hearing Disorders

Interpretation of the audiogram, including determining type of hearing impairment, was discussed in Chapter 4. In the current chapter, examples of audiograms associated with common hearing disorders are demonstrated. Examples of common conductive hearing losses are depicted in the first section, consistent with otitis media, otosclerosis, ossicular chain discontinuity, and cholesteatoma. Two-ear audiograms are shown with all audiograms displayed in this chapter and symbols appear in black and white. The student is reminded also to gain experience with audiograms where the two ears are displayed on one audiometric grid. Masked symbols may or may not be seen on the audiogram, depending on the need for performing masking. One recalls that conductive hearing losses typically display a loss by air conduction (AC), normal bone conduction (BC) thresholds, and presence of significant air-bone gaps (ABGs). In re-examining the rules for masking by both AC and BC, it is readily apparent that masking will probably be performed with conductive losses, to obtain accurate BC thresholds. On occasion, the audiologist must also perform masking to ensure that AC thresholds are valid. The maximum degree of hearing impairment with a purely conductive hearing loss is approximately 60 to 65 dB HL and the audiologist

159

should bear in mind that a medical referral is in order as the hearing loss is often reversible.

Although this textbook concentrates on pure-tone audiometry, such testing rarely occurs in isolation within the audiology clinic. As pure-tone findings are described with each disorder, the student gains practice in integrating all other aspects of the comprehensive evaluation: case history, speech audiometry, immittance audiometry, special tests, and recommendations. As a general rule, the speech recognition thresholds (SRTs) should be in good agreement with pure-tone averages (PTAs). Word Recognition Scores (WRS) generally will be quite good to excellent with conductive hearing losses. Immittance audiometry typically will yield abnormal tympanograms and acoustic reflex measurements. Following the generation of the audiogram, the audiologist is prepared to counsel and make appropriate recommendations. As the disorder is present within the outer and/or middle ear, remediation strategies most probably will involve medical and/or surgical intervention.

Otitis Media

Otitis media or middle ear infections are among the most frequently diagnosed childhood diseases in the United States, especially during the first few years of life. Approximately 70% of children experience at least one episode of acute otitis media (AOM) before the age of three years (Jordan & Roland, 2000). Otitis media accounts for one-third of medical visits in childhood and millions of annual emergency room visits, as well as approximately 25% of oral antibiotic prescriptions (Castagno & Lavinsky, 2002). Anatomically, one of the primary precursors is dysfunction of the eustachian tube, which normally serves to aerate and equalize pressure within the middle ear space. Children are more predisposed as their eustachian tubes are shorter and more horizontally placed than those of older children and adults, although the disease may also occur in adulthood. Bacteria present in the nasopharynx spread to the middle ear, where they replicate and cause infection. The eustachian tube may also become swollen and infected, leading to inhibition of its normal functions. If the eustachian tube remains chronically closed, negative pressure will develop within the middle ear, resulting in a retracted tympanic membrane and presence of fluid or effusion (Roland, 1995).

High-risk factors include enrollment in daycare, exposure to secondhand smoke, craniofacial anomalies, family history, chronologic age of eight years or under, and membership in at-risk ethnic groups. Prevalence is higher between the ages of 6 to 24 months, in males, among patients with allergies, during certain seasons, and among Caucasian, Native American, and Eskimo populations (Jordan & Roland, 2000). Signs and symptoms may include irritability, fever, pulling or tugging at the ears, history of middle ear infection, sleeplessness, loss of appetite, and otalgia. Upon otoscopic examination, the audiologist may note redness and inflammation of the ear canal and tympanic membrane (TM). The audiologist may further note a bulging or retracted TM, TM dullness and discoloration, perforation, and/or presence of effusion (Castillo & Roland, 2007). Chronic infection may demonstrate long-term effects on the tympanic membrane, with repeated retraction causing thinning and stretching of the membrane. If the retracted TM rests on the incus, ossicular erosion and/or discontinuity could result, as well as a moderate conductive hearing loss. Recurrent infections may also lead to hyalin deposits on the TM surface, leading to tympanosclerosis, although such deposits do not greatly affect hearing sensitivity (Roland, 1995).

Figure 9–1 shows a typical audiogram that may be seen clinically with an otitis media patient. Although otitis media is often present bilaterally, it also may occur unilaterally. In this case, the hearing loss is bilaterally symmetric and of a mild degree, most probably a result of presence of effusion and limited TM mobility. Note that AC thresholds demonstrate the mild hearing impairment that slightly rises in configuration from 250 to 8000 Hz. Although it is not uncommon for masked AC thresholds to be noted with a conductive hearing loss,

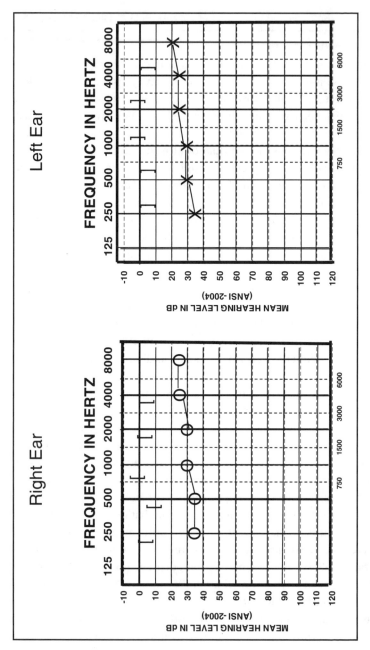

Figure 9–1. Sample audiogram for otitis media patient.

masking was not necessary in this case. According to Hunter and colleagues (1994), AC hearing sensitivity may be best at 2 kHz, with elevated thresholds seen in lower and higher frequencies. BC thresholds in the example audiogram are within normal limits from 250 to 4000 Hz bilaterally and masking was necessary with all, in view of significant air-bone gaps. Masking levels noting the plateau obtained should be recorded on the audiogram.

Upon medical referral, medication may be recommended although courses of antibiotics are not as prevalently recommended as they have been historically. In chronic cases, the patient may undergo surgical intervention in the form of myringotomy with placement of tympanostomy tubes. As with any medical disorder, audiologic monitoring following medical/surgical treatment is necessary. The audiologist plays a major role in pre- and postoperative audiologic evaluations, as well as regular tympanostomy tube checks. Presence of otitis media may result in daily fluctuating hearing impairment, with even mild losses resulting in speech, language, and/or academic difficulty. Counseling and a team approach is essential, especially in the case of a preschool or school-aged child. Complications of chronic, untreated otitis media may include TM perforation, mastoiditis, tympanosclerosis, cholesteatoma, and intracranial infections such as meningitis.

Otosclerosis

Otosclerosis is a disease that involves excessive resorption of bone, followed by growth of abnormal bone tissue (Jerger & Jerger, 1981). It appears to be more common in females than in males and often manifests itself during pregnancy. The abnormal bone tissue, soft at first and then sclerotic in later stages, most often is located at the stapes footplate of the middle ear. Etiology is unclear, although it is theorized that there may be infectious, genetic, vascular, or other contributing factors. It is often bilateral and familial, although unilateral cases have been reported, as have mixed hearing losses. Figure 9–2 shows a pure-tone audiogram that was obtained from a patient with otosclerosis.

Although the hearing loss is asymmetric, note that the type is conductive in both ears. With conductive hearing losses, significant ABGs may not be noted at each frequency; in addition, significant ABGs may exist and must be noted, even when AC thresholds may appear within normal limits. With this audiogram, AC thresholds for the right ear indicate primarily a mild to moderate degree of hearing loss, whereas AC thresholds for the left ear indicate a milder impairment rising to normal limits. Pure-tone averages of 37 dB HL and 23 dB HL are noted for the right and left ears, respectively, using the three-frequency method of calculation. In applying previously delineated masking rules, it was not necessary to mask any AC thresholds for this patient. As is typical with conductive hearing losses, BC thresholds were masked in view of significant ABGs and are within normal limits. One classic audiometric manifestation with otosclerosis is a "Carhart notch," first described in 1952 (Carhart, 1952). This involves a notch or depressed BC threshold in the frequency region of 2 kHz and most probably is a result of mode of intertial BC loss and/or a shift in normal middle ear resonance (Margolis & Goycoolea, 1993). Rappaport and Provencal (2002) suggested that the Carhart notch disappears following surgery and that it is related to resonance of the external ear canal and fixed ossicular change.

During case history elicitation, this patient may report familial history of hearing loss and that his or her own loss is gradually progressive. One ear may or may not be subjectively better in sensitivity. Otoscopic examination may be unremarkable, although an occasional Schwartze's sign is noted. This sign is characterized by a TM rosy glow, resulting from a promontory area that has become highly vascularized (Martin & Clark, 2009). As with any conductive impairment, a team approach is necessary in diagnosis and in implementation of remediation strategies. Extensive counseling is required regarding audiologic results and recommendations. Patients may undergo a

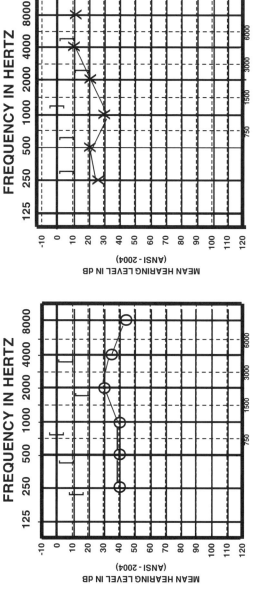

Figure 9–2. Sample audiogram for otosclerosis patient.

variety of treatments, including medication for attempting to arrest the disease process and/or surgical intervention to ameliorate the stapes fixation. Best practice includes baseline testing with pure-tone audiometry prior to medical/surgical treatment and close monitoring following treatment. Although a medical referral is a primary clinical course of care and although conductive loss patients are typically not hearing aid candidates, an occasional patient may be "at risk" for surgical intervention. These patients may seek amplification on medical clearance and may benefit greatly, in view of wide dynamic ranges, excellent word recognition abilities, and other factors.

Ossicular Chain Disarticulation/Discontinuity

Patients may experience ossicular chain discontinuity at any age, with common causes being infection, head trauma, barotrauma, foreign body, or other types of injury. The injury results in disruption of normal articulation of ossicles and related physiology. The conductive hearing loss is often sudden and unilateral, with key information provided via case history. In children, the most common cause of ossicular discontinuity is necrosis resulting from otitis media, causing the incudostapedial connection to become fibrous (Roland, 1995). In addition to important case history information, results of otoscopic examination also are important with ossicular discontinuity patients. In the case of trauma, the audiologist may see ear canal abrasions and/or also may note hemotympanum, or an accumulation of blood behind the tympanic membrane (TM). Figure 9–3 demonstrates an audiogram seen with a young adult male patient, following a motor vehicle accident where trauma occurred to the right side.

AC thresholds for the left ear are well within normal limits from 250 to 8000 Hz with an essentially flat audiometric configuration, other than at 8 kHz. For the right ear, however, a moderate to mild conductive hearing loss is noted. AC thresholds for the right ear fall within the mild to moderate hearing loss range with a flat configuration.

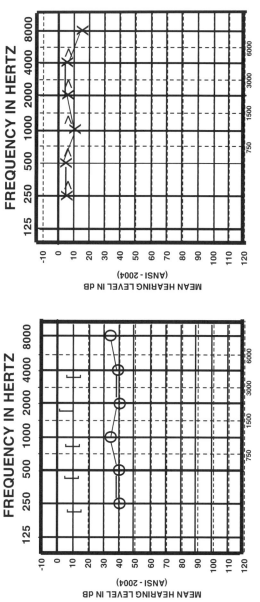

Figure 9–3. Sample audiogram for ossicular discontinuity patient.

167

Pure-tone averages of 38 dB HL and 7 dB HL may be calculated for the right and left ears, respectively. When discontinuity occurs as a result of fibrous replacement of bone, as may be observed with otitis media, the ABGs may be more prevalent in the higher frequencies of the audiogram.

In integrating pure-tone audiometry with other components of a comprehensive audiologic test battery, the audiologist should note that trauma patients may also experience dizziness and associated sensorineural hearing loss. In such cases, immediate surgical intervention may be in order to repair any perilymph fistula, or opening that may have occurred between the middle and inner ear spaces. Medical referral is in order whenever ossicular discontinuity is suspected, in order to confirm diagnosis and to seek treatment options. Often, surgical intervention is the treatment of choice to restore ossicular articulation and normal function whenever possible. Previous surgeries may also result in discontinuity of the ossicular chain. For example, patients with history of cholesteatoma may have experienced a bony destruction process prior to surgical removal. The medical team, including the audiologist, should attend to concomitant complaints such as otalgia, nausea, dizziness or lightheadedness, and others. As with any patient, thorough counseling and proper follow-up are mandatory.

Cholesteatoma

Patients experiencing chronic or untreated otitis media may experience a host of complications such as TM perforation, mastoiditis, chronic drainage, and cholesteatoma (Chole & Forsen, 2002). Cholesteatoma is defined as a false tumor made up of dead epithelial tissue and other debris that has collected within the middle ear cavity. It may be acquired or congenital, at times developing with no apparent cause. Conductive hearing loss from cholesteatoma typically is slowly developing, although the loss may progress more rapidly in the presence of infection. The degree of hearing loss, if present, may be dependent on location of the debris accumulation within the tympanum or epitympanum. Primary symptoms are otalgia, progressive conductive hearing loss, unresponsiveness to medical treatment, chronic drainage, and otorrhea or abnormal odor. Cholesteatomas are typically unilateral, although bilateral ones may be evident. Although this "false tumor" is typically benign, the bolus of material is slowly growing and eventually must be removed, as with any such growth housed in such close proximity to the brain.

Obtaining of a thorough case history is important, as with any disorder, with red flags including the chronic drainage and unresponsiveness to treatment at any age. A medical team approach toward case management is essential, with cholesteatoma patients serving as frequent visitors to audiology and otolaryngology clinics. Upon otoscopic examination, the audiologist may view the cholesteatoma, depending on its size and location either behind the TM or even extruding from the TM. Figure 9–4 reveals a sample audiogram obtained with presence of a cholesteatoma in the left ear. Audiologic and otolaryngologic examination of the right ear is within normal limits.

AC testing for the right ear reveals hearing sensitivity well within normal limits from 250 to 8000 Hz with no significant air-bone gaps observed. For the left ear, a mild to moderate conductive hearing loss is seen, slightly falling in audiometric configuration. AC thresholds for that ear are outside the normal range, whereas masked BC thresholds are within normal limits from 250 to 4000 Hz. Significant air-bone gaps are observed for the left ear. PTAs of 8 dB HL and 35 dB HL are noted for the right and left ears, respectively.

Although pure-tone audiometry is the focus of this text, the audiologist interprets these findings in conjunction with all other aspects of the comprehensive test battery. With many conductive hearing losses, medical and/or surgical treatment may alleviate the hearing impairment and "close" or eliminate the significant air-bone gaps. The primary purpose of cholesteatoma management is to treat any infection medically and often to surgically remove the tissue growth.

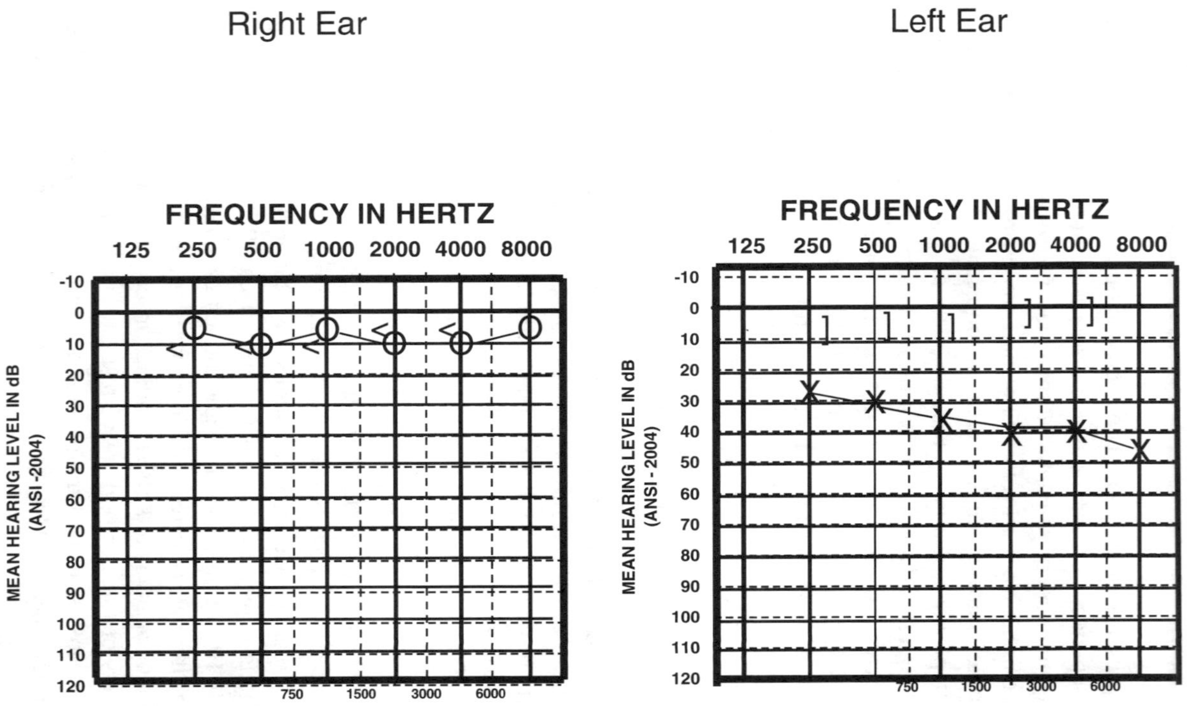

Figure 9–4. Sample audiogram for cholesteatoma patient.

In certain instances, infected material may erode middle ear structures and also affect hearing physiology. Cholesteatoma patients must undergo extensive counseling and follow-up, in the event of recurrence. Because a residual unilateral hearing impairment may be present following treatment, the audiologist may implement rehabilitative strategies for unilateral hearing loss: amplification, communication strategy training, hearing assistive technology, ongoing monitoring, preferential seating, and other measures. As with most conductive hearing loss patients, amplification on medical clearance may be successful, in this case with careful management of chronic drainage.

Many additional external and/or middle disorders exist and are seen routinely in the audiology clinic, other than the illustrations presented above. Further examples of external and/or middle ear disorders include otitis externa, atresia, anotia, foreign bodies, and various types of tissue or bony growths (Chole & Forsen, 2002). Typically, many of these entities do not result in conductive hearing loss unless the ear canal is occluded. Cerumen impaction, if not removed prior to testing, may result in conductive hearing loss. Collapsed ear canals also may reveal conductive hearing impairment on the audiogram, if insert earphones are not utilized. The audiologist also may see other types of middle ear disorders that may result in conductive hearing loss, including eustachian tube dysfunction, genetic hearing loss, childhood syndromes, and congenital anomalies.

SENSORINEURAL HEARING LOSS

The audiologist also clinically evaluates many patients who suffer from disorders that result in sensorineural hearing loss (SNHL). Perhaps two of the most common disorders are presbycusis, or hearing loss as a result of aging, and noise-induced hearing loss. Case history is an important aspect of the diagnostic battery and medical referral often indicated, although medical and/or surgical treatment generally is not effective in restoration of hearing. Many SNHL patients are prime candidates for aural (re)habilitation, that may include hearing aid evaluation, cochlear implantation, speech reading, auditory training, speech and/or language intervention, hearing assistive technology, and other strategies.

Pure-tone audiometry provides the audiologic foundation, with AC and BC thresholds each demonstrating hearing loss that may range from slight to profound in degree. No significant air-bone gaps are noted and a variety of audiometric configurations may be seen. In integrating all test findings with pure-tone results, the clinician should see SRTs within good agreement of the PTAs. Contrary to findings with conductive hearing losses, the WRS may range from excellent to poor. Performance on WRS testing may be directly correlated with magnitude of hearing impairment and audiometric configuration has great effect on target phoneme discrimination. Tympanometry is expected to be within normal limits, with acoustic reflex testing results dependent on effect of pathology along the acoustic reflex arc. Many patients with cochlear hearing losses also exhibit recruitment or abnormal loudness growth, a phenomenon that must be taken into consideration during the amplification process.

Presbycusis

Patients with presbycusis comprise a large component of the clinical audiologist's patient population, especially with advanced medical care and increased life expectancy in this country. Schuknecht and Gacek (1993) described six different types of presbycusis including sensory, neural, strial or metabolic, cochlear conductive, mixed, and intermediate. In eliciting case history information, the clinician should recall that disorder effects may be cumulative throughout a life span; that is, a number of causes may have contributed to a patient's hearing loss. The classic presbycusic audiogram shows a mild to moderate, falling configuration that is sensorineural in type. Greatest degree of hearing loss appears in frequencies above 1 kHz. Although the loss is usually bilateral and symmetric, great variability may be seen in magnitude and configuration. Changes due to aging may occur in the middle ear, inner hair cells, and central auditory pathways. Patients may demonstrate cochlear degeneration with progressive axonal, ganglion cell, or hair cell loss (Mazelova, Popelar, & Syka, 2003). An example of an audiogram obtained on an 82-year-old female patient may be seen in Figure 9–5.

AC and BC pure-tone thresholds are superimposed and this hearing loss is of a mild to moderate degree, gradually falling in configuration. PTAs in this case are 30 dB HL and 32 dB HL for the right and left ears, respectively. Responses to both pure-tone and speech stimuli may be delayed with elderly patients and speech audiometric findings may be poorer than pure-tone findings indicate. On occasion, monitored live voice testing may be necessary for all speech measures because presbycusic patients may not be able to respond to taped stimuli in a timely manner.

Following comprehensive audiologic evaluation, extensive counseling is in order and family members are often involved in evaluation, counseling, and rehabilitative processes. Presbycusis patients, including the one whose audiogram is illustrated in Figure 9-5, typically are hearing aid candidates as well as candidates for other rehabilitative strategies. Other forms of hearing assistive technology also may be beneficial. Challenges may be present with regard to the hearing aid selection process, such as narrow dynamic range, poorer than expected word recognition abilities, limited finances, transportation difficulties, manual dexterity issues with regard to hearing aid controls, and cognitive decline. The audiologist should exercise compassion and empathy in treating the "whole person." The audiologist should also bear in mind that the patient may be at increased risk of falling from vestibular disorder, may have been prescribed numerous medications, and may be under a physician's care for a variety of other medical problems.

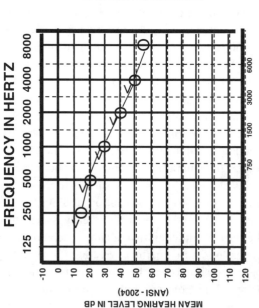

Figure 9–5. Sample audiogram for presbycusis patient.

174

Ménière's Disease

Audiologists who work within a medical setting see numerous adult patients who suffer from Ménière's disease. Although precise etiology is unknown, this debilitating disorder is thought to result from the body's abnormal production and/or reabsorption of endolymph. Swelling of endolymphatic spaces of the inner ear may occur within the cochlea and/or the semicircular canals of the vestibular system. The cause may be related to overproduction of endolymph by the stria vascularis or by underabsorption due to failure of the endolymphatic sac (Schuknecht, 1975). Obtaining of case history information is crucial, in that patients present with a classic triad of symptoms that include fluctuating hearing loss, bothersome tinnitus, and debilitating vertigo. In addition to fluctuating, the hearing impairment is typically unilateral and the patient also often experiences aural fullness.

Reliable pure-tone testing may be challenging in patients with tinnitus, in that false-positive responses may be seen. Strategies for obtaining the most accurate possible thresholds include presenting warble or pulsed tone stimuli and/or presenting initial stimuli at suprathreshold levels, so that the patient is familiarized with the stimulus. AC testing generally reveals a unilateral, sensorineural hearing loss in one ear that fluctuates from test session to test session. This disorder is one of the few that displays a rising audiometric configuration. Figure 9–6 demonstrates a sample audiogram of a Ménière's disease patient whose right ear is affected by the disorder.

In the right ear, a moderate rising to mild sensorineural hearing loss is noted in the presence of normal to borderline normal hearing sensitivity for the left ear from 250 to 8000 Hz. BC testing reveals absence of significant air-bone gaps in either ear, confirming the sensorineural type of hearing impairment in the right ear. Pure-tone averages of 40 dB HL and 17 dB HL are seen in the right and left ears, respectively.

Degree of hearing loss in the affected ear is likely to progress along with progression of the disease. In addition to a comprehensive

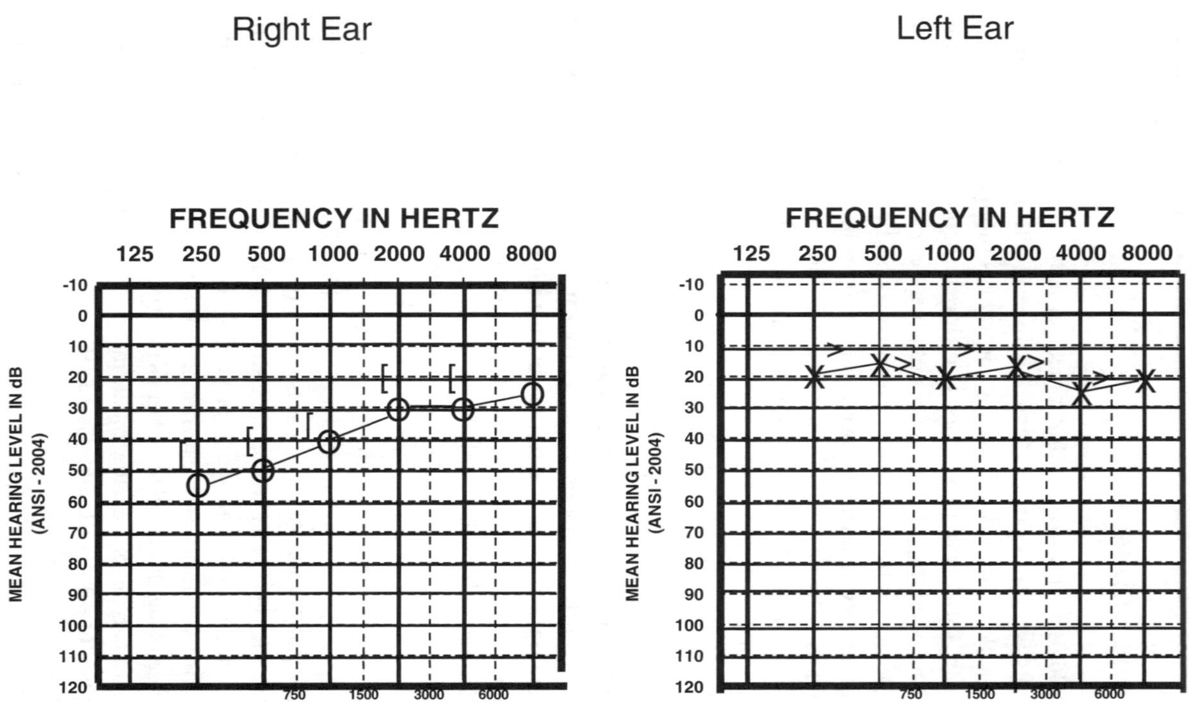

Left Ear

Right Ear

Figure 9–6. Sample audiogram for Ménière's disease patient.

audiologic evaluation, the audiologist may also see this patient for vestibular function tests such as video-oculography, rotary chair, computerized posturography, and vestibular evoked myogenic potentials. Electrophysiologic measures may also be performed; electrocochleography, especially, has been beneficial in helping to diagnose Ménière's disease. Patients also may be referred for imaging studies, such as computerized axial tomography (CT scan) or magnetic resonance imaging (MRI). A team approach of medical professionals is indicated, as always, with exercising of compassion as patients are often noting dizziness, nausea, vomiting, and other uncomfortable complaints (Castillo & Roland, 2007). Empathetic counseling is a standard of quality care with possible treatment options being: dietary management, medications to address symptoms and/or serve as diuretics, and even surgical intervention in some cases. Hearing aid fitting as a rehabilitative strategy for the unilateral, sensorineural hearing loss is a possible option in some cases. Advances in the form of digital programming and digital signal processing are advantageous when addressing a hearing impairment that may exhibit daily fluctuations. Finally, some Ménière's disease patients have been candidates for cochlear implantation on progression of the disease and hearing loss, pending hearing sensitivity in the unaffected ear.

Ototoxicity

Occasionally, a patient may be prescribed medications that are ototoxic. These medications, often administered in the presence of life-threatening illnesses, may potentially damage cochlear and/or vestibular structures. The poisonous effects of the toxin may result in temporary or permanent hearing loss and/or vestibular dysfunction (Roland & Marple, 1997). The audiologist's role is to remain current regarding the list of ototoxic medications, examples of which include chemotherapeutic agents, aminoglycoside antibiotics, antimalarial medications, loop diuretics, quinine, and high doses of aspirin (Campbell, 2007). The audiologist works closely with medical personnel and especially with physicians who are prescribing the medications and determining dosages. As many monitoring patients are inpatients, the audiologist becomes familiarized with hospital room bedside and intensive care unit audiologic procedures. Many patients may be too ill to transport to the audiologic suite and/or too ill to adapt to required audiologic tasks for long time periods.

Whenever possible, it is important to obtain baseline audiometric thresholds prior to treatment administration; a monitoring schedule is established, with thresholds obtained on an ongoing and regular basis, throughout the course of treatment. As described in Chapter 7, serial audiogram forms are often utilized for this purpose so that thresholds may readily be compared. Because threshold changes are more likely to occur in the ultrahigh-frequency region, high-frequency audiometry is an important complement to the thorough audiologic evaluation performed at conventional test frequencies. The audiologist may notify the physician of significant change in hearing thresholds, after which a dosage and/or medication alteration may be possible prior to affecting the more traditional "speech" frequencies. It should be noted that this alteration is not always possible, nor is it always possible to maintain hearing status in the presence of medication for such serious illness. Figure 9–7 shows an example of a traditional audiogram for a patient who experienced severe hearing loss as a result of ototoxic medication. Thresholds beyond 8 kHz are not noted.

The audiometric configuration appears to be symmetric and slightly falling, bilaterally. PTAs of 80 dB HL are observed bilaterally with absence of significant ABGs. In this case, many BC thresholds are beyond the equipment limits and the sensorineural hearing loss may be confirmed via other methods, such as history, medical examination, and immittance audiometry. With respect to speech audiometric measures, poor WRS would also be expected bilaterally. The clinician extends empathy and compassion while extensively counseling the patient and family regarding audiologic results and

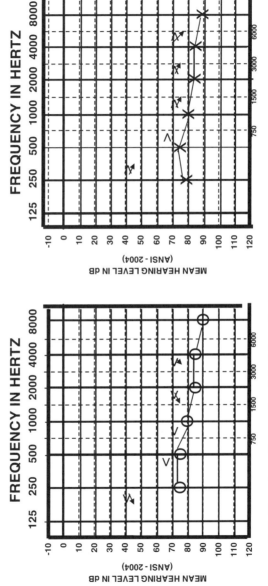

Figure 9–7. Sample audiogram for ototoxicity patient.

179

recommendations. While bearing in mind that medical difficulties are extensive and complex, the audiologist may recommend various remediation strategies on stabilization of the medical condition. These may include vestibular rehabilitation, hearing aids, communication training, referral to the cochlear implant team, ongoing follow-up, and many others to enhance quality of life. Referral to a cochlear implant team may be a viable option for the patient whose audiogram is demonstrated in Figure 9–7.

Noise-Induced Hearing Loss

Noise-induced hearing loss (NIHL) is the second most common sensorineural hearing loss, with 10 million Americans currently suffering hearing impairments caused by frequent exposure to hazardous noise levels (Clark & Bohne, 1999). Patients may experience either temporary or permanent shifts in auditory thresholds. Audiologists play a great role in hearing conservation and prevention of noise-induced hearing impairment. Industrial audiologists become familiar with Occupational Safety and Health Administration (OSHA) Standards and monitor both the work environment and the hearing of industrial workers. In addition to work-related noise, patients may suffer from hearing loss as a result of recreational noise such as target shooting, serving in the military, and many other variations. Noise-induced hearing loss is typically progressive and symmetric, affecting the higher frequencies. The hearing impairment may be accompanied by tinnitus, with the patient reporting that he can "hear but not understand what is said." Patients also often have difficulty communicating in group settings and within noisy environments. Harmful effects are dependent on noise intensity, duration, frequency spectrum, and individual patient susceptibility.

The audiogram demonstrates a sensorineural hearing loss, as a result of cochlear damage, often with a notched configuration most apparent from 3 to 6 kHz. The exact location of the notch depends on numerous factors, including ear canal dimensions and frequency spectrum of the damaging noise (Clark, 2008). On occasion, the hearing impairment may be asymmetric, for example, in the case of target shooting, hunting, or acoustic trauma affecting one ear over the other. Excessive noise exposure may damage outer hair cells by metabolic exhaustion and/or structural damage such as fused stereocilia and broken tip links. Inner hair cell innervations may be disrupted via swelling or splitting of afferent terminals (Clark, 2008). Figure 9–8 exhibits a sample audiogram, obtained with a construction worker who has been exposed to occupational noise for approximately 20 years.

In both ears, hearing sensitivity is within normal limits to borderline normal, with the exception of a notch at 4 kHz to the moderate hearing loss range. The loss is slightly asymmetric at 2 kHz, falling to the mild hearing loss range at that frequency for the right ear. The audiologist receives important clues regarding noise exposure history from the referral source, testing circumstances, and case history information. During pure-tone testing, false-positive responses may be noted if tinnitus is present; frequency-modulated and/or pulsed tones may be implemented, in addition to other testing strategies previously described for tinnitus patients. With regard to the current audiogram, a PTA of 10 dB HL is obtained for the right ear with usage of the two-frequency calculation method. Recall that the two-frequency method is used when a 20 dB or more difference exists between consecutive frequencies implemented in the PTA calculation. When the two-frequency method is indicated, the audiologist selects the better two frequencies for averaging. A PTA of 12 dB HL is calculated for the left ear, with use of the traditional three-frequency method. Mid-octave frequencies are tested for the right ear at 1.5 and 6 kHz for the right ear and at 3 and 6 kHz for the left ear, in view of the large threshold differences seen between adjacent octave frequencies. Bone conduction testing reveals absence of significant air-bone gaps and substantiates that the hearing loss is sensorineural in type.

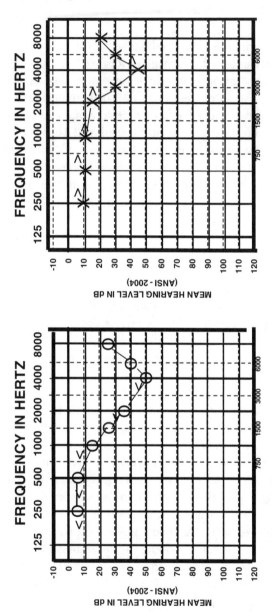

Figure 9–8. Sample audiogram for patient with noise-induced hearing loss.

182

The audiologist would expect the WRS to fall within the good to excellent range, with the patient experiencing discrimination confusions of high-frequency consonant phonemes. Because these high-frequency sounds are crucial toward speech intelligibility and may be missed in conversation, it is apparent that connected speech may sound unclear even though the listener may actually hear that it is present. Patients exposed to excessive noise should be counseled regarding prevention strategies that include reducing exposure to the dosage, wearing of ear protection, and other measures. As with ototoxic monitoring, a baseline audiogram is important prior to noise exposure and regularly throughout the history of noise exposure. Industrial audiologists may obtain thresholds with several patients simultaneously, utilizing previously described automatic audiometric techniques, or may evaluate via more traditional methods. Extensive counseling should be implemented, especially if threshold shifts are seen, with audiologist and patient noting possible cumulative effects of noise, medication, aging, and other disorders. As with any patient with sensorineural hearing impairment, rehabilitative strategies may include hearing aids, communication strategies training, hearing assistive technology, and others.

These cases highlight only several of the many different hearing disorders that may lead to sensorineural hearing impairment. Other causes may include childhood syndromes, nonsyndromic forms of genetic hearing loss, bacterial meningitis, congenital maternal infections, trauma, and a variety of additional etiologies (Mencher et al., 1997). Sensorineural hearing loss may be acquired or congenital, manifesting in either a gradually progressive or sudden manner. In some cases, the loss is idiopathic with unknown cause. With this second type of hearing impairment, the audiogram displays AC thresholds that may be slight to profound in magnitude. Although the configuration may vary widely, this audiometric shape and the symmetry parameter provide valuable clues regarding etiology. BC thresholds are superimposed with AC thresholds, revealing absence of significant ABGs, consistent with a normally functioning outer and middle ear system. Masking may be needed for AC and/or BC if a great enough asymmetry is present between the two ears.

Audiograms depicting mixed hearing losses, the third type of hearing impairment, have appeared in Chapter 4. The reader recalls that these cases involve a combination of conductive and sensorineural pathology with the following demonstrated on the audiogram: hearing loss seen when viewing both AC and BC thresholds and significant ABGs. There are many possible combinations of conductive and sensorineural pathologies; for example, a mixed hearing loss may be seen on the audiogram with a child who exhibits a sensorineural hearing loss from meningitis and who is experiencing a bout of otitis media. An additional example is a presbycusic patient who is suffering from a large TM perforation and consequent conductive component on the audiogram.

CENTRAL DISORDERS

Acoustic Neuroma

In addition to helping to identify and remediate hearing disorders that occur within the peripheral auditory system, the audiologist also works closely with patients who experience disorders of the central auditory nervous system. One such disorder is an acoustic neuroma, also known as a vestibular schwannoma. This is typically a benign, slowly-growing tumor that occurs within the region of the VIIIth cranial nerve and can affect hearing and/or vestibular function. Hearing loss may occur as the blood supply to the cochlea is compromised (Selesnick & Jackler, 1992). As the tumors continue to grow, exerted pressure may also affect other cranial nerves and the brainstem. Although the neuroma may occur bilaterally, it is most often unilateral. Prior to the advent of electrophysiologic and imaging measures, acoustic neuromas were quite large when first identified. As described in Chapter 10, the audiologist historically performed a site-of-lesion test battery, many tests of which relied heavily on pure-tone stimuli, for helping to identify the central or retrocochlear pathology. With the advent of new technology, however, the audiologist and other medical team members are often able to identify the neuroma in its earlier stages. Figure 9–9 shows an audiogram of an adult patient who was newly identified as suffering from a small acoustic neuroma on the right side. Case history information may provide crucial diagnostic clues and may include such complaints as unilateral tinnitus, hearing loss, disequilibrium or imbalance, facial numbness or weakness, or distorted speech perception on the affected side. In later stages, patients may report such entities as visual disorder, gait disturbances, headaches, and other symptoms associated with central disorder (Jackler & Pfister, 2005). Hearing loss typically begins in the higher frequencies, occasionally demonstrated as a sudden loss that also may be fluctuating.

In the unaffected left ear, one may note that AC thresholds are well within normal limits from 250 to 8000 Hz. For the affected right ear, however, one notes hearing sensitivity within normal to borderline normal limits, with a slightly falling configuration. Of great significance is the asymmetry seen in higher frequencies from 2 to 8 kHz. PTAs of 8 dB HL and 7 dB HL are observed for the right and the left ears, respectively. Bone conduction testing reveals absence of significant air-bone gaps.

On integrating pure-tone audiometry with other test findings, one may expect a lower word recognition score (WRS) than pure-tone thresholds might indicate. This finding is a "red flag" for indication of central pathology, as is presence of word recognition "rollover," defined as a significant decrease in the WRS at high presentation intensity levels. The immittance audiometry battery also may provide important clues to the audiologist regarding suspicion of acoustic neuroma. Specifically, elevated or absent acoustic reflexes may be seen on the affected side. Significant acoustic reflex decay also may be present. Standard protocol would be to perform ABR with this patient,

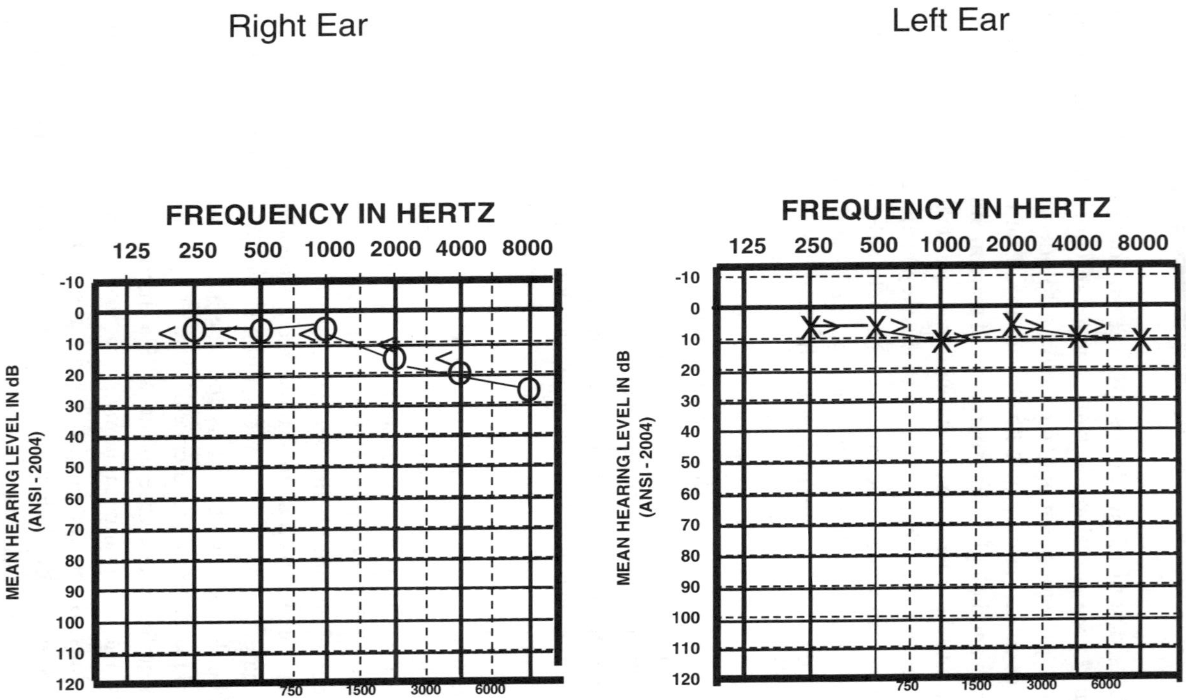

Figure 9–9. Sample audiogram for patient with acoustic neuroma.

with expectation of abnormal tracings on the right side (Mencher et al., 1997). Magnetic resonance imaging (MRI) would be performed prior to scheduling the patient for surgical intervention, often the treatment of choice when an acoustic neuroma is diagnosed. With small tumors, the physician may adopt a "wait and see" plan, although eventual tumor removal is likely. During the surgical procedure, the audiologist may play a key role with regard to intraoperative monitoring (IOM) via electrophysiologic techniques. Although the initiation of IOM has led to increase in neural function preservation, many patients experience postoperative unilateral deafness due to compromised neural function. In these cases, the audiologist also plays an important role with respect to postoperative audiometry, amplification, and other rehabilitative techniques.

Auditory Neuropathy

Auditory neuropathy (AN), also known as auditory dyssynchrony, is a relatively newly discovered disorder that may manifest itself in many different audiometric magnitudes and configurations. The hearing loss, when present, is often sensorineural and of a significant magnitude, as shown in Figure 9-10. Many risk factors for AN are similar to those that place a child at risk for significant hearing loss, including such entities as low birthweight, hereditary factors, and hyperbilirubinemia. Although the etiology of AN is complex and much has yet to be discovered, location of the disorder is thought to lie more central to the outer hair cells of the cochlea (Starr, Picton, Sininger, Hood, & Berlin, 1996). AN patients have historically also experienced marked difficulty with speech perception, to a greater degree than pure-tone findings may indicate. Hearing loss as demonstrated by pure-tone findings may fluctuate.

With regard to the sample audiogram, AC thresholds indicate a moderately severe to mild/moderate sensorineural hearing loss bilaterally, rising in configuration. PTAs of 50 dB HL and 57 dB HL

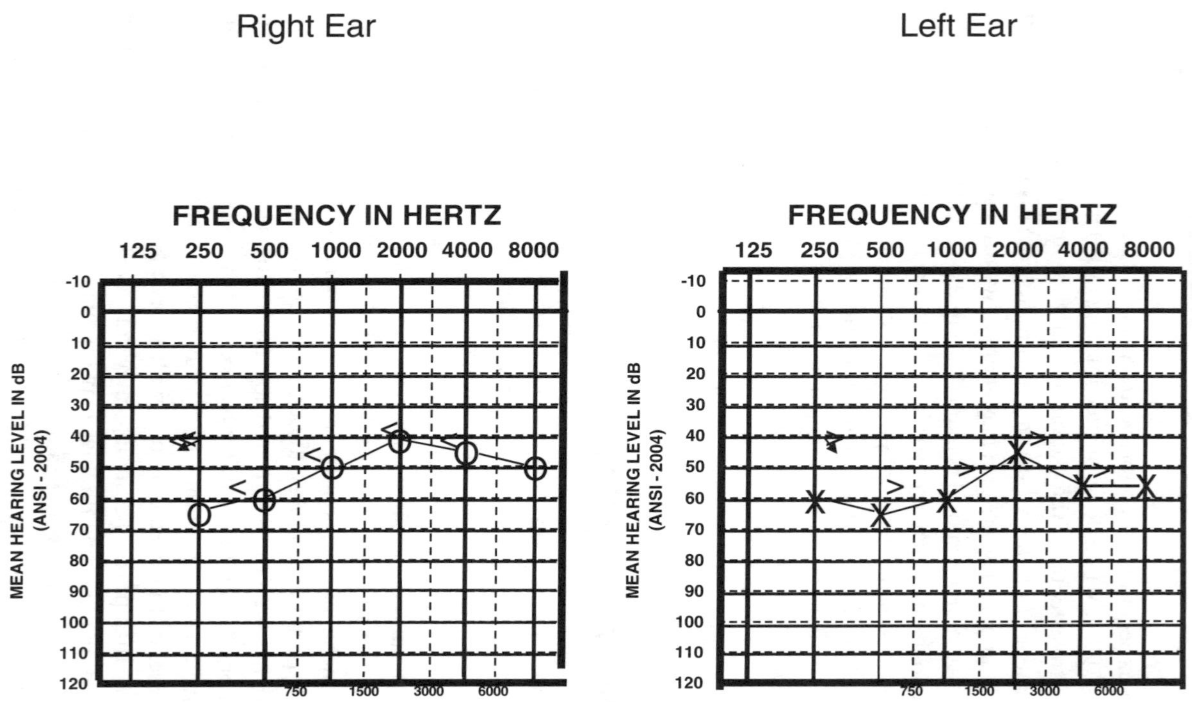

Right Ear

Left Ear

Figure 9–10. Sample audiogram for patient with auditory neuropathy.

are calculated for the right and left ears, respectively. Performance of speech audiometry will be challenging in view of speech perception difficulty; word recognition scores will be poor, in all likelihood, especially through use of auditory cues alone. Acoustic reflex patterns will probably reflect abnormalities present along ipsilateral and/or contralateral reflex arc pathways.

A combination of OAEs and ABR testing traditionally has been performed in many cases and as part of a larger test battery, for differential diagnosis. In cases of AN, OAEs often are present in light of normal outer hair cell function and in the presence of abnormal ABR tracings. Aural (re)habilitation strategies, crucial and highly dependent on individual patient communicative needs, may include many of those already discussed for sensorineural hearing loss such as amplification, hearing assistive technology, alternate modes of communication, and communication strategy training. In some cases and when the patient is a candidate for cochlear implantation, the device has served to enhance neural synchrony and led to communication benefits (Trautwein, Sininger, & Nelson, 2000).

Auditory Processing Disorders (APD)

Auditory processing disorders may be present across the life span, from school-aged children through elderly populations. Auditory processing may be described as perceptual processing of auditory information in the central nervous system, with a disorder referring to adverse effect on this process (Bellis, 2007). Patients with APD may demonstrate a variety of symptoms that include distractibility in noise, difficulty understanding complex directions, discrimination difficulty among sounds, and difficulty comprehending auditory information. The audiologist plays a major role in diagnosis of APD, in conjunction with a team approach, utilizing many complex tests that involve degradation of the signals and taxing of the auditory system. The first step in evaluation is performance of a pure-tone audiogram, an example of which is provided in Figure 9–11.

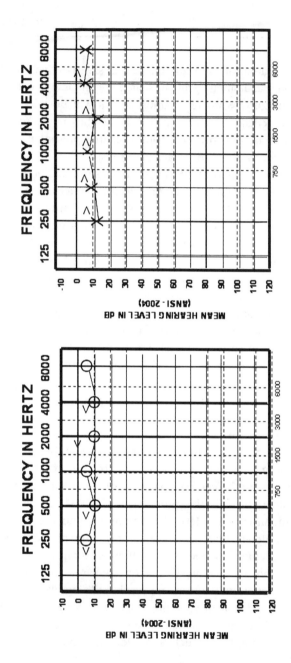

Figure 9–11. Sample audiogram for patient with auditory processing disorder.

Many individuals with APD demonstrate normal hearing sensitivity on the audiogram, although some patients with peripheral hearing impairment are diagnosed with APD. As one views the sample audiogram, one notes that AC thresholds are within normal limits bilaterally from 250 to 8000 Hz. PTAs of 8 dB HL are calculated bilaterally, via a three-frequency method. BC thresholds are also within normal limits bilaterally from 250 to 4000 Hz with no significant ABGs seen. Word recognition abilities may be poorer than pure-tone findings indicate, especially in the presence of noise, and performance diminishes with challenging listening tasks. The audiologist also plays a major role in remediation that may include enhancement of the signal-to-noise ratio, auditory training, other forms of communication training, teacher in-servicing, and modification of the acoustical environment.

The final three audiograms displayed here have illustrated only three of many disorders affecting the central auditory nervous system (CANS). Additional disorders such as trauma, the aging process, vascular disease, autoimmune disease, and numerous others also may affect anatomic structures and physiology of the CANS. The audiology student is encouraged to further study the myriad hearing disorders affecting the peripheral and/or central auditory mechanisms, as well as the manner in which they are displayed on the audiogram. With heightened experience, the audiologist sharpens audiogram interpretation skills. He or she, in turn, becomes competent in utilizing the crucial information obtained via pure-tone audiometry and other aspects of the test battery toward identification of hearing impairment and applying optimum strategies toward the highest quality of hearing health care.

REFERENCES

Bellis, T. J. (2007). Historical foundations and the nature of (central) auditory processing disorder. In F. E. Musiek & G. D. Chermak (Eds.), *Handbook of (central) auditory processing disorder: Auditory neuroscience and diagnosis* (Vol. 1, pp. 119–136). San Diego, CA: Plural.

Campbell, K. C. M. (2007). Pharmacology in audiology. In R. J. Roeser, M. Valente, & H. Hosford-Dunn (Eds.), *Audiology diagnosis* (pp. 157–168). New York: Thieme Medical.

Carhart, R. (1952). Bone conduction advances following fenestration surgery. *Transactions of the American Academy of Ophthalmology and Otolaryngology, 56,* 621–629.

Castagno, L. A., & Lavinsky, L. (2002). Otitis media in children: Seasonal changes and socioeconomic level. *International Journal of Pediatric Otolaryngology, 62,* 129–134.

Castillo, M. P., & Roland, P. S. (2007). Disorders of the auditory system. In R. J. Roeser, M. Valente, & H. Hosford-Dunn (Eds.), *Audiology diagnosis* (pp. 77–99). New York: Thieme Medical.

Chole, R. A., & Forsen, J. W. (2002). *Color atlas of ear disease* (2nd ed). Hamilton, Ontario, Canada: B. C. Decker.

Clark, W. W. (2008). Noise induced hearing loss. In W. W. Clark & K. K. Ohlemiller (Eds.), *Anatomy and physiology of hearing for audiologists* (pp. 321–340). New York: Thomson Delmar Learning.

Clark, W. W., & Bohne, B. (1999). Effects of noise on hearing. *Journal of the American Medical Association, 281,* 1658–1659.

Hunter, L. L., Margolis, R. H., & Giebink, G. S. (1994). Identification of hearing loss in children with otitis media. *Annals of Otology, Rhinology and Laryngology, 103,* 59–61.

Jackler, R. K., & Pfister, M. H. F. (2005). Acoustic neuroma (vestibular schwannoma). In R. K. Jackler, & D. E. Brackmann (Eds.), *Neurotology* (2nd ed., pp. 727–782). Philadephia: Mosby.

Jerger, S., & Jerger, J. (1981). *Auditory disorders: A manual for clinical evaluation.* Boston: Little, Brown & Company.

Jordan, J. A., & Roland, P. S. (2000). Disorders of the auditory system. In R. J. Roeser, M. Valente, & H. Hosford-Dunn (Eds.), *Audiology diagnosis* (pp. 85–108). New York: Thieme Medical.

Margolis, R. H., & Goycoolea, H. G. (1993). Multifrequency tympanometry in normal adults. *Ear and Hearing, 14,* 408–413.

Martin, F. N., & Clark, J. G. (2009). *Introduction to audiology* (10th ed.). Boston: Pearson.

Mazelova, J., Popelar, J., & Syka J. (2003). Auditory function in presbycusis: Peripheral and central changes. *Experimental Gerontology*, *38*, 87–94.

Mencher, G. T., Gerber, S. E., & McCombe, A. (1997). *Audiology and auditory dysfunction*. Boston: Allyn & Bacon.

Rappaport, J. M., & Provencal, C. (2002). Neuro-otology for audiologists. In J. Katz (Ed.), *Handbook of clinical audiology* (pp. 9–32). Baltimore: Lippincott Williams & Wilkins.

Roland, P. S. (1995). Medical aspects of disorders of the auditory system. In R. J. Roeser & M. P. Downs (Eds.), *Auditory disorders in school children* (pp. 57–75). New York: Thieme Medical.

Roland, P. S., & Marple, B. F. (1997). Disorders of inner ear, eighth nerve and CNS. In P. S. Roland, B. F. Marple, & W. L. Meyerhoff (Eds.), *Hearing loss* (pp. 195–258). New York: Thieme Medical.

Schuknecht, H. F. (1975). Pathophysiology of Ménière's disease. *Otolaryngologic Clinics of North America*, *8*, 507–514.

Schuknecht, H. F., & Gacek, M. R. (1993). Cochlear pathology in presbycusis. *Annals of Otology, Rhinology, and Laryngology Supplement*, *102*, 1–16.

Selesnick, S. H., & Jackler, R. K. (1992). Clinical manifestations and audiologic diagnosis of acoustic neuromas. *Otolaryngology Clinics of North America*, *25*(3), 521–551.

Starr, A., Picton, T. W., Sininger, Y., Hood, L. J., & Berlin, C. I. (1996). Auditory neuropathy. *Brain*, *119*, 741–753.

Trautwein, P. G., Sininger Y. S., & Nelson, R. (2000). Cochlear implantation of auditory neuropathy. *Journal of the American Academy of Audiology*, *11*, 309–315.

10 *Pure-Tone Audiometry: Past, Present, and Future*

The evolution of traditional pure-tone audiometry has been previously described, as has its significance in serving as an important diagnostic foundation. Pure-tone stimuli have also played a major role with regard to additional historical and current diagnostic measures. Prior to the advent of electrophysiology and its use in differential diagnosis, the audiologist composed a test battery for identification of central pathology. Following are brief descriptions of some of the measures utilizing pure-tone stimuli, as well as the phenomena on which they are based. As audiologists developed a central auditory nervous system (CANS) battery, it was important to utilize "battery" as an operative word and not to interpret any one test in isolation.

Békésy Audiometry

Békésy audiometers were commonly noted about the audiology clinic prior to arrival of current technology, which includes electrophysiologic measures (Békésy, 1947). These audiometers typically were of an automatic variety, whereby the patient was instructed to press a button as long as a continuous or pulsed tone was heard and to release the button when the tone became inaudible. Pure-tone thresholds could be ascertained via tracings, in either a discrete or continuous frequency manner. Figure 10–1 shows a sample tracing obtained via automatic audiometry. A downward excursion indicates that the signal is becoming louder; when the patient presses the button indicating the stimulus is heard, the excursion moves in an upward direction and the intensity level decreases. When the patient releases the button on no longer hearing, the stimulus increases in intensity. This cycle repeats itself as threshold is traced. Threshold may be viewed as the excursion midpoint at a particular frequency, in conjunction with a threshold definition of softest audible level at least 50% of the time.

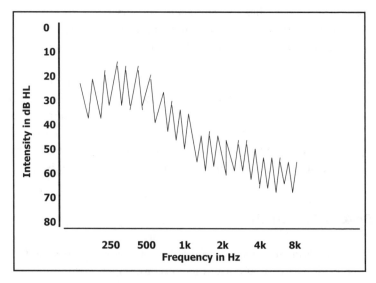

Figure 10–1. Example of an automatic audiometry tracing.

In addition to bracketing threshold for determining hearing sensitivity, Békésy tracings were helpful in distinguishing cochlear from central lesions. Two threshold tracings were obtained for the affected ear, in a sweep-frequency fashion: one utilizing pulsed pure-tone stimuli and one utilizing continuous stimuli. The theory on which the test was constructed is based on abnormal adaptation. That is, with a central disorder, the neural firing should maintain while pulsed tone thresholds are being traced. However, abnormal adaptation may likely occur during continuous tonal threshold tracings, causing these tracings to fall either significantly below those of pulsed-tone thresholds or to the limits of the equipment. Pulsed and continuous tonal tracings should be superimposed, for the most part or at least within specific limits of one another, for those lesions that are not of central etiology.

Tone Decay

Tone decay testing also utilizes pure-tone stimuli of various frequencies and is based on an abnormal adaptation phenomenon that may be present with central disorder (Carhart, 1957; Hood, 1955). The task involves presenting a continuous tone at a suprathreshold level, and asking the patient to respond as long as he or she hears the tone. Various methods have involved testing at differing intensity levels, with most common being +5 dB SL and +20 dB SL (with reference to pure-tone threshold at that frequency). If a central disorder exists and abnormal adaptation is present, the patient initially should respond and then cease to respond on fatigue. Upon ceasing to respond, the intensity of the tone is increased by 5 dB; although a patient with a central disorder may newly respond, the tone may rapidly fade once again and require an additional intensity increase. The amount of tone decay is reported in dB, calculated as the audiologist compares final with beginning presentation levels of the tone. With peripheral disorders, the patient should either maintain the continuous tone for an extended period of time or exhibit a minimal amount of tone decay. Procedures have also varied with regard to length of tonal presentation time. Some audiologists have recorded for a total of 60 seconds whereas others have sought a full 60-second positive response, restarting the stopwatch on every negative response.

Short Increment Sensitivity Index (SISI)

Although Békésy audiometry and tone decay testing were based on the abnormal adaptation premise, other tests such as the Short Increment Sensitivity Index (SISI) were based on the phenomenon of abnormal loudness growth (Jerger, Shedd, & Harford, 1959). Recruitment has been defined as an abnormal growth in loudness perception and most often is seen with cochlear pathology.

Pure-tone stimuli for this and other tests within the "CANS" battery have often been presented to the affected ear from 500 to 4000 Hz. With the SISI, a training session is conducted prior to test administration. The patient hears a continuous tone presented at 20 dB SL (with reference to pure-tone threshold at that frequency), with an occasional and random 5 dB intensity increment. The patient is instructed to respond by button-pushing on hearing the "jump in loudness." Once this task is mastered, the training session then involves the same task with the intensity increment lowering to a 3 dB increase in loudness. The actual test incorporates presenting the continuous tone with 20 randomly interspersed, 1 dB increments in loudness above the continuous tone. The patient is to respond each time he or she hears the very small increase.

As may be expected, patients with cochlear pathology who experience abnormal loudness growth are more likely to perceive the small, 1 dB loudness increment. The audiologist keeps track of positive responses out of the 20 presentations, with each positive response contributing 5% to a total possible score of 100%. Patients with recruitment achieve high scores, whereas patients with central pathology will likely not hear the small increment resulting in a low score. Interpretation difficulties arise with scores that are neither clearly indicative of recruitment nor clearly indicative of absence of recruitment.

Alternate Binaural Loudness Balancing (ABLB)

Alternate Binaural Loudness Balancing (ABLB), also based on the phenomenon of recruitment, was performed when an asymmetry of approximately 20 dB or more existed between ears at any one frequency. This test was first described by Fowler in 1928 and was performed when the poorer ear was suspected of central pathology. Pure tones of the same frequency are presented alternately at a specified presentation level above pure-tone threshold (20 dB SL, for example). With the better ear serving as a reference, the task is to vary the intensity level in the poorer ear until loudness matching is subjectively reported by the patient. The task is repeated at louder intensity levels, for example, in 20 dB increments until a "laddergram" is obtained comparing loudness perception in one ear with that of the other. Several different outcomes are possible. The first is that there could be a linear and equal growth of loudness in both ears. Second, there could be a normal loudness growth in the better ear with an abnormal growth in the poorer, such that a specified dB HL level eventually is perceived as being equal in loudness despite the original inequality in thresholds. A third possible outcome is that the growth in loudness and resultant dynamic range of the affected ear becomes abnormally wide as opposed to abnormally narrow. With regard to interpretation, the reader should bear in mind that such tests have been performed to discern cochlear from central disorder; presence of recruitment in this case was indicative of cochlear findings whereas absence of recruitment was indicative of noncochlear pathology.

Monaural Loudness Balancing (MLB) involves a similar loudness-matching task between different frequencies of the same ear, when an asymmetry of 20 dB or more exists between their thresholds. Test administration and interpretation are similar to those described for the ABLB, with presence of recruitment being a critical variable in determining cochlear from central disorder.

The above tests may have been part of a "CANS" battery when history or comprehensive audiologic evaluation was suggestive of central pathology. Primary causes for suspicion were poorer than expected WRS, unexplained pure-tone asymmetry, elevated or absent acoustic reflex thresholds (unanticipated in light of pure-tone findings), and presence of acoustic reflex decay. Acoustic reflex decay testing represents another important clinical use of pure-tone stimuli. With its performance, a tonal stimulus is presented at a suprathreshold level for 10 seconds. Significant diminishing of the reflex amplitude may be an indication of central pathology. The audiologist also may have performed WRS rollover testing within the realm of speech audiometry. In this case, a Performance Intensity-Phonetically Balanced (PI-PB) function was conducted in the form of full word recognition word lists at intensity levels above traditional levels. WRS were assessed in 10 dB or 20 dB increments past routine levels for WRS testing. With abnormal adaptation and fatigue often seen with central disorder, the WRS may become increasingly and significantly poorer at higher presentation levels. The audiologist quanitified presence or absence of significant rollover via formulae that took into consideration maximum and minimum WRS.

Positive battery findings often resulted in medical referral that included radiologic studies. With the advent of Auditory Brainstem Response (ABR) testing and other electrophysiologic measures, many of the site-of-lesion diagnostic measures are no longer performed. Upon noting of "red flags" via case history or audiologic evaluation, the typical clinical course currently is toward referral for ABR and MRI.

PEARLS AND PITFALLS: CURRENT PURE-TONE AUDIOMETRIC TECHNIQUES AND MASKING

Preparation for Testing

Prior to performance of pure-tone testing, the audiologist typically elicits important case history information. Many clinicians devise case history forms for both adult and child populations, as they develop expertise in eliciting the most relevant information within an efficient time period. Because a finite time period exists for each patient visit, the examiner must skillfully delve into pertinent areas, while maximizing the time and focusing on items that are most relevant. As opposed to asking "yes"/"no" questions from a checklist, the audiologist may merely ask "What can you tell me about your hearing?" The individual's story is likely to unfold at this point, requiring periodic probing on the examiner's part. Similarly, the pediatric audiologist may ask "What can you tell me about your child's hearing?" perhaps making a few relevant inquiries prior to the test session and completing the interview post-testing while the child is allowed to play. Furthermore, the clinician must extract accurate information in a compassionate and empathetic manner, with ease at handling difficult topics. A streamlined procedure, particularly geared toward time constraints and sensitive discussion points, is to request that the history form be completed prior to the appointment time. The audiologist's patient load may involve culturally and linguistically diverse populations. This requires the professional to be experienced with communication among various cultures, perhaps seeking use of an interpreter during case history interviewing, counseling, and pretest instructions. Word lists for speech audiometry may be available for those patients for whom English is a second language.

Otoscopic examination is completed prior to beginning pure-tone testing, often one of the first diagnostic measures performed.

The experienced clinician must become well versed regarding landmarks observed during the otoscopic examination, red flags for immediate medical referral, and disorders that may be observed within the outer and/or middle ear. Many audiologists are highly skilled at cerumen management, when deemed necessary prior to testing.

Familiarity and comfort with audiologic equipment and new technology is a must within the audiology practice. The audiologist is prepared well in advance for the patient visit, having calibrated according to ANSI standards and performed daily listening checks. The audiologist should remain current with regard to new equipment technology, standards, and procedures. He or she should invest in equipment required for calibration and feel comfortable progressing through all required steps. In addition to extensive reading regarding proper calibration and other equipment maintenance protocols, the audiology student should master techniques with hands-on experiences and strive toward lifelong learning.

Pure-Tone Testing Session

Most students begin audiology practice with fellow students, utilizing conventional techniques with adult patients who may be in good health and whose responses are highly consistent. Upon transition toward a variety of clinical settings, however, the student rapidly learns that there are challenging-to-test patients with whom standard, conventional techniques may be ineffective. The beginning audiologist gains skill and knowledge related to equipment and testing procedures. As he or she derives a greater depth of experience, clinical insight is developed toward accurate test administration and insightful interpretation of results. Each patient and clinical situation is truly individualized and techniques must be adapted for each diagnostic session. The audiologist is fortified with knowledge regarding various hearing/vestibular disorders and other medical conditions, carrying out a team approach in treating the whole person. Each step of the testing session dictates what additional steps will be taken. For example, there may be a reason for not testing the better ear first or for progressing through test frequencies in a nontraditional manner. A patient may be reluctant to push a button or raise a hand in responding, causing the audiologist to create a different reliable response mode. It is very important that the audiologist be able to determine presence or absence of response from outside the test suite, where equipment is located. In interpreting responses, the examiner considers the required response along with many other forms of body language, utilizing all available resources for the most accurate possible AC and BC thresholds.

When attention span of the patient is limited, the audiologist may seek only 2 of 4 positive responses at one frequency as the 50% criterion, before progressing to the next. When responses are seen at the softest intensity limit of the equipment, the modified Hughson-Westlake procedure may itself require modification. For example, if the softest limit is −10 dB HL and the patient responds at −5 dB HL, the audiologist will not be able to descend by 10 dB following the positive response. With patients exhibiting severe-to-profound losses or no responses at the high intensity limits of the equipment, the audiologist who typically begins testing within the 40 dB HL range may save time by starting at a higher intensity level. As the audiologist gains an even greater level of experience, clinical insights will allow pre-evaluation educated guesses regarding configurations, types of losses, approximate mid-octave thresholds, speech audiometric results, and other measures. Whenever AC thresholds are symmetric and significant ABGs are absent, the audiologist may choose to perform BC testing with transducer placement on only one ear. These results represent unmasked BC thresholds, with masking deemed unnecessary.

The audiologist may deal with additional interesting behaviors, besides those of positive versus negative response to the pure-tone stimulus. It is important to be able to communicate with the patient via a talk-back system and to monitor stimuli presented. Reinstruction is often necessary, as is gently reminding the patient of tasks required. The patient's well-being, comfort, and medical condition should be continually monitored. One example of an unusual testing situation may be a patient who is claustrophobic on closing the audiometric suite door. This fear may be alleviated with counseling, opening the door on occasion, keeping the door slightly open if within a quiet room, or facing the patient chair toward the examiner window. A second example of an unusual testing behavior is the patient who falls asleep during testing, as the examiner continues to raise the intensity dial in 10 dB steps. The patient may be refocused by verbal reinstruction, presentation of a slightly louder stimulus, providing a testing break, or the examiner's physically reentering the room to refocus the patient's attention. A third example is the patient who continually narrates what he is hearing, informing the tester that he hears nothing, whereas that tone is louder and that one seems very remote. This patient must be reminded to remain very quiet, lest he miss one of the very faint tonal stimuli. The reader, audiology students and practicing clinicians may think of endless other examples. With practice and experience, the pure-tone threshold obtaining and masking procedures become automatic with assurance of reliable results with each individual patient.

Although the masking process is one of the most difficult encountered by the student of Audiology, learning is solidified through practice and hands-on experiences. As with most aspects of audiology practice, one must first learn theory and techniques academically prior to bridging toward clinical application. A common progression with mastering of masking is to answer the "why" and "when" questions prior to learning "how." As one practices masking rule application with sample audiograms, these concepts transition toward the patient who demonstrates significant ABGs or audiometric asymmetry. As confidence and clinical intuition develop, the audiologist visualizes when masking is necessary as the pure-tone audiogram evolves. Setting up of equipment, determination of tonal and narrow-band noise levels, the actual procedure, and recording of results become rewardingly automatic. Audiologists implement masking according to a variety of procedures, although all are seeking the same outcome of achieving minimum to maximum effective masking and accurate thresholds. Some patients adapt readily to masking tasks whereas others find it difficult to continue to listen for the tone while disregarding the noise. The astute and patient audiologist reinstructs and works with his or her patients toward understanding of tasks required. If the patient is unable to adapt to masking tasks, the audiologist may note this on the audiogram form and seek desired information in additional ways of checks and balances throughout the test battery. For example, immittance audiometry results help to provide information about middle ear status if presence of significant ABGs is in question.

Interpretation of the audiogram is another difficult concept for the student of Audiology. Some slight variation exists among members of the profession regarding constitution of a significant ABG, although determining type and magnitude of hearing impairment appears somewhat standardized. Upon consulting different audiologists, one may learn that determination of symmetry and configuration patterns appears to be less rule-driven and more variable. As pure-tone thresholds are ascertained and results recorded on the audiogram, the audiologist should continually be exercising detective work regarding possible disorder and next steps toward the evaluation process. As emphasized in Chapter 1, pure-tone audiometry is a cornerstone of the diagnostic evaluation, providing crucial information on its own merit and serving as a springboard for further evaluative measures. Rarely performed in isolation, the pure-tone audiogram must be created and interpreted in conjunction with other comprehensive evaluative measures: speech audiometry and immittance audiometry. Case history, medical/physical examination, otoscopic examination, and any previous testing results contribute to a vast armamentarium of knowledge regarding the patient. Similarly, the audiologist assimilates all pieces leading up to and including the pure-tone audiogram, so as to make additional diagnostic recommendations that may be in order: ABR, vestibular evaluation, OAEs, imaging studies, medical specialty referral, psychoeducational referral, and countless other possibilities.

Upon completion of pure-tone audiometry, the audiologist must immediately be prepared to counsel the patient regarding the audiogram and other comprehensive audiologic findings. Explanations must be clear and geared toward the individual patient and family members. Remediation strategies are discussed, such as referral to other disciplines, hearing aid evaluation, hearing assistive technology, communication training, educational recommendations, and a host of other options.

Report Writing

Although the audiologist often writes a brief line or two of interpretation on the audiogram form, it is important to develop full report-writing skills. Such formal reports are geared toward the intended audience, beginning with patient identifying information and a case history summary. Professional writing style of the case history section includes referring to self in the third person and alleviating irrelevant information that does not relate to patient complaints. Facts should be reported in an objective manner. Areas that may not be verified should be presented with an "According to the patient/parent . . . " preface. The audiologist should attain all previous audiograms and additional records whenever possible, bearing in mind that his or her own records must be accurate and thorough. In addition to report writing, it is crucial to document all patient contacts, visits and related communications so that a "paper trail" is available regarding all aspects of the patient's care.

Although report styles vary, one viable format is to create three paragraphs under the "Audiologic Evaluation Results" heading: one describing pure-tone findings, a second to describe speech audiometric findings, and a third to describe immittance audiometry. Further paragraphs may describe additional test results and impressions, although the audiologist should avoid making medical diagnoses. Recommendations are listed in the final section of a professional report.

Within the "Audiologic Results Section" the writer may begin to describe pure-tone findings in the first paragraph by noting audiologic techniques utilized and his or her own subjective reliability rating. Assuming an adult patient, the report may progress as follows with adaptations made toward other populations: an introductory statement conveys techniques used for pure-tone testing and the clinician's assessment of reliability of results. The writer should present all parameters of audiogram interpretation: magnitude, symmetry, configuration, and type. This information is possible to convey in one sentence, as proper flow and conciseness develop with clinician practice and experience. It is important to consider the entire frequency range when interpreting parameters, and not merely the PTAs or speech frequencies. The reader should be able to visualize the audiogram by simply reading the written description. In the presence of asymmetry, two sentences are necessary for thorough description. For example, a sentence may describe one ear with normal hearing sensitivity from 250 to 8000 Hz and another sentence may describe a moderate, flat sensorineural hearing loss. Research findings supporting the AMCLASS validated tool for classifying audiograms may also provide helpful information to the clinician during counseling and report writing (Margolis & Saly, 2008). Specifically, the authors describe distribution of hearing loss characteristics in a large clinical sample. Such findings allow the audiologist to compare an individual's audiogram with configuration, type, magnitude, and site-of-lesion prevalence of a larger population.

It is important to state the PTAs, in that these will be compared to SRTs in a subsequent paragraph. In finalizing the first paragraph that summarizes pure-tone findings, the writer should compare current with previous audiogram results. One may then state whether significant changes were seen since the time of the last evaluation on a specified date. If significant changes were noted, it is important to state this finding, frequencies where changes were noted, and the amount of decrease or increase. It is not necessary to discuss masking; rather, it is understood that masking was appropriately performed when necessary for AC and/or BC thresholds and that the interpretations are made through viewing of the true thresholds. Masked symbols are noted on the audiogram, where applicable, and implemented noise levels are recorded.

Although this textbook focuses on pure-tone audiometry, it is critical for the audiologist to integrate the audiogram with other test findings. Subsequent paragraphs of a report should present results of speech and immittance audiometry. Interpretation is critical, following reporting of results and scores. If test scores are presented with no interpretation, the reader may be at a loss as to meaning.

ADDITIONAL UTILIZATIONS OF PURE-TONE STIMULI

Characteristics of sound, such as measurement of frequency in Hz and intensity in dB, are fundamental toward understanding sound and its use in comprehensive audiologic evaluation. Pure-tone signals serve as integral components of psychoacoustics, the study of how various parameters of sound are perceived by a listener.

Differential sensitivity, although not often performed clinically, has held relevance in research and hearing science. Through usage of a reference and a varied pure-tone stimulus, Just Noticeable Differences (JNDs) or Difference Limens (DLs) may be determined. Specifically, the second tone may be varied with regard to basic parameters of frequency, intensity, and/or time and compared to the first tone (with which the parameters remain constant). Small increments of such basic parameters are implemented until the point where the listener subjectively judges that the two signals are different, as opposed to the same. For example, a judgment may be that "tone B is just noticeably higher (lower) in pitch, just noticeably louder (softer), or just noticeably longer (shorter) than tone A." Similarly, two or more tonal stimuli may be presented for ascertaining matching tasks, whereby the two tones are perceived as equal in pitch, loudness, or duration. Psychophysical scales have also traditionally existed in the hearing science literature, involving a task where a variable pure-tone stimulus is compared to a reference one. For example, the mel scale is one whereby pitch judgments, such as a "doubling of pitch" or "halving of pitch" are made between tonal frequencies. The sone and phon scales have existed to plot subjective loudness judgments between two tonal stimuli: the former with regard to "doubling or halving the loudness" with progression from one stimulus to the next and the latter with regard to generation of equal loudness contours across frequency. Equal loudness contours may be obtained across the dynamic range, from threshold of audibility to very high intensity levels. Each point along a specific contour is considered to be equal in loudness, with variability seen from frequency to frequency.

Other important uses of pure-tone stimuli within the research and hearing science arenas have included, for example, tasks for demonstrating benefit of binaural listening. Localization tasks have been performed utilizing pure- or warble-tone stimuli, as well as for demonstration of the binaural summation effect where binaural threshold is approximately 3 dB more acute than monaural threshold. Phase and intensity differences of pure-tone and other stimuli, as they arrive at the two ears, have proven responsible for release from masking when a listener communicates within a noisy environment. Finally, pure-tone stimuli have helped to demonstrate the head shadow effect with monaural listeners, as the far ear is in the "shadow" of the head when stimuli are presented to the near ear. Lower frequency stimuli with longer wavelengths are more likely to diffract around the head in this case, whereas higher frequency stimuli with shorter wavelengths are more likely to be reflected away from the head. Clearly, and as demonstrated by these examples, pure-tone stimuli have often served as stimuli of choice with regard to hearing science research, discovering important information about disordered versus normal processes, and supplying a solid foundation for clinical work.

As has been emphasized, pure-tone audiometry serves as the cornerstone for the comprehensive audiologic evaluation although it does not stand alone. Its usage is to determine frequency-specific AC and BC thresholds so that the clinician may interpret parameters of type, configuration, symmetry, and magnitude of hearing loss. The pure-tone audiogram is integrated with other test findings, such as speech and immittance audiometry. Furthermore, it is assimilated with any other diagnostic measure that may be performed. On occasion, AC thresholds may be obtained in isolation; for example, this may occur when regular monitoring is taking place. Additional uses of pure-tone stimuli within diagnostic audiology are many, some of which have been previously described within this text.

Audiologists work closely with patients who suffer from tinnitus and occasionally utilize pure-tone stimuli to "match" frequency and intensity characteristics of those stimuli with the individualized tinnitus. Electrophysiologic measures, such as ABR testing, OAEs, Electrocochleography (ECoG), Middle Latency Response (MLR), Late Evoked Responses (LER), and other forms of evoked potentials, may be performed utilizing brief tone bursts or tone pips as stimuli. As previously described, many of these measures are objective, utilized for such purposes as helping to estimate threshold or assisting in the differential diagnosis process. Although techniques and protocols vary, tonal stimuli are typically presented from 500 to 4000 Hz. Within the vestibular evaluation arena, Vestibular Evoked Myogenic Potentials (VEMPs) may also utilize brief tone bursts as auditory stimuli for elicitation of the response. Waveforms elicited are thought to originate from the saccule and serve to complement other test findings: rotary chair, computerized platform posturography, video-oculography, and others.

The audiologist also finds pure-tone audiometry useful with the selection and verification of hearing aids and other amplification systems. For example, either pure-tone or speech stimuli may be utilized to determine Most Comfortable Loudness Levels (MCLs) and Loudness Discomfort Levels (LDLs). The individual frequency information secured via pure-tone audiometry is especially useful in fitting devices comfortably within patients' dynamic ranges. With regard to electroacoustic analysis of hearing aids, FM systems, and other hearing assistive technology, sweep pure-tone stimuli play a major role. Specifically, frequency response curves demonstrate gain, output, and other measures as a function of frequency and are crucial toward attaining a high-quality fitting. With regard to verification, unaided and aided warble tone thresholds traditionally have been assessed within the sound field at various frequencies, in order to assess functional gain. This technique of viewing unaided and aided thresholds is also being implemented to help the audiologist assess cochlear implant benefit. State-of-the-art equipment and techniques allow real-ear probe microphone verification by comparing real-ear unaided with real-ear aided responses, in determination of real-ear gain. These gain curves once again display gain and output as a function of sweep frequency.

Other examples of pure-tone stimuli uses within diagnostic audiology are found within the auditory processing evaluation, most commonly performed with school-aged children and sometimes performed with adults. Many different types of tasks that tax the auditory system are present within the battery, including measurement of such skills as temporal processing, dichotic listening, auditory closure, sequencing, and auditory figure-ground. Although some tests carry a high linguistic load, it is also important to select tests that carry a lighter linguistic load in the event of speech and/or language disorder. Pure-tone stimuli are key with regard to those tests that carry a lighter linguistic load and are not composed of speech stimuli. Furthermore, the audiologist selects evaluative instruments appropriate for patient age that tap into various auditory skills and differing components of the central auditory nervous system.

Although many tests for auditory processing disorder (APD) utilize speech audiometry in the form of single words or sentences, others are based on pure-tone audiometry. The Pitch Pattern Sequence Test involves presentation of tonal stimuli that are composed of two different frequencies: 880 Hz and 1122 Hz (Pinheiro & Ptacek, 1971; Ptacek & Pinheiro, 1971). These tones are presented in groups of three, and the reader is to respond as to the "high" or "low" pitch pattern. The Duration Pattern Sequence Test involves presentation of tonal stimuli that are equal in frequency, but of two different durations: 250 msec and 500 msec (Pinheiro & Musiek, 1985). These tones are presented in groups of three, and the reader is to respond as to the "long" or "short" temporal pattern. Poor performance with these tests may indicate difficulty with frequency and/or temporal processing, respectively, and may point to a cerebral lesion (Musiek & Pinheiro, 1987). A third example of an APD test that may be based on pure-tone stimuli is the Masking Level Difference (MLD), although the MLD may also be measured with use of speech stimuli. As a first step in MLD measurement, a tonal threshold is obtained in noise with absence of phase or temporal differences (Hirsch, 1948; Licklider, 1948). After phase shifting, a second tonal threshold is obtained in the presence of noise. If phase and intensity difference cues are being properly assimilated within the brainstem, the second threshold should be lower and more sensitive than the first. The difference in decibels between the two thresholds is called the MLD. If no improvement is seen and the MLD is very small, APD or other central pathology may be suspected. It is evident through these examples that pure-tone stimuli are extremely useful with regard to basic audiometric measures and more sophisticated measures across the life span and across audiology's scope of practice. Clinical masking is not limited to the pure-tone audiogram. The audiologist should perpetually be aware of rules for AC and BC masking, performing masking with any procedure if the possibility exists of crossover to the nontest ear.

FUTURE TRENDS

With explosion of new technology, it is an exciting time to be a member of the Audiology profession. Audiologic equipment will become more and more advanced and computerized, along with continued miniaturization of components. Efforts are being exerted toward a validated system that categorizes audiometric configuration, severity and site-of-lesion. This AMCLASS™ system may prove beneficial in categorizing audiograms for research purposes, providing validated interpretation to enhance treatment approaches, facilitating communication regarding audiologic findings, and promoting the student's learning regarding audiogram interpretation (Margolis & Saly, 2007).

It is evident that pure-tone audiometry historically has played a major role in identification of hearing impairment, that it currently plays a major role, and that it will continue to play a major role. Future trends, along with advanced technology, may be incorporation of more automatic techniques rather than manual pure-tone audiometry. Enhanced simulations via technology may help the beginning audiologist with such difficult tasks as calibration, audiogram interpretation, and masking. More standardized procedures may be developed so that audiologists implement similar protocols with masking and determination of hearing loss configuration, symmetry, type and magnitude. The audiologist's experience and expertise will always be needed, despite technology and automated procedures, for keen insight regarding patient response, interpretation of test results, recommendations relative to further diagnostic measures, extensive counseling, and planning of remediation strategies.

REFERENCES

Békésy, G. v. (1947). A new audiometer. *Acta Otolarygologica, 35*, 411-422.

Carhart, R. (1957). Clinical determination of abnormal adaptation. *AMA Archives of Otolaryngology, 65*, 32-39.

Fowler, E. P. (1928). Marked deafened areas in normal ears. *Archives of Otolaryngology, 8*, 151-155.

Hirsh, I. J. (1948). The influence of interaural phase on interaural summation and inhibition. *Journal of the Acoustical Society of America, 20*, 536-544.

Hood, J. D. (1955). Auditory fatigue and adaptation in the differential diagnosis of end-organ disease. *Annals of Otology, Rhinology, and Laryngology, 64*, 507-518.

Jerger J., Shedd, J. L., & Harford, E. (1959). On the detection of extremely small changes in sound intensity. *Archives of Otolaryngology, 69*, 200-211.

Licklider, J. C. R. (1948). The influence of interaural phase relations on the masking of speech by white noise. *Journal of the Acoustical Society of America, 20*, 150-159.

Margolis, R. H., & Saly, G. L. (2007). Toward a standard description of hearing loss. *International Journal of Audiology, 46*, 746-758.

Margolis, R. H., & Saly, G. L. (2008). Distribution of hearing loss characteristics in a clinical population. *Ear and Hearing, 29*(4), 524-532.

Musiek, F. E., & Pinheiro, M. L. (1987). Frequency patterns in cochlear, brainstem and cerebral lesions. *Audiology, 26*, 79-88.

Pinheiro, M. L., & Musiek, F. E. (1985). Sequencing and temporal ordering in the auditory system. In M. L. Pinheiro & F. E. Musiek (Eds.), *Assessment of central auditory dysfunction: Foundations and clinical correlates* (pp. 219-238). Baltimore: Williams & Wilkins.

Pinheiro, M. L., & Ptacek, P. H. (1971). Reversals in the perception of noise and tone patterns. *Journal of the Acoustical Society of America, 49*, 1778-1782.

Ptacek, P. H., & Pinheiro, M. L. (1971). Pattern reversal in auditory perception. *Journal of the Acoustical Society of America, 49*, 493-498.

Glossary

Acoustic Reflex Thresholds (ARTs): part of the immittance audiometry battery, this refers to the softest intensity level at which the acoustic reflex may be measured

Air-Bone Gap: significant difference between air conduction and bone conduction thresholds in the same ear at any particular frequency

Air Conduction (AC): method of testing with earphones, insert earphones or loudspeakers such that the signal is delivered through the entire hearing mechanism, including the periphery and central auditory nervous system

American National Standards Institute (ANSI): organization that devises and publishes standards required for various test procedures and protocols

Audiogram: graph displaying hearing sensitivity, showing Frequency in Hz across the x-axis and Intensity in dB along the y-axis

Audiometer: piece of equipment used by the audiologist to evaluate hearing sensitivity

Auditory Brainstem Response (ABR) Testing: electrophysiologic measure utilized by audiologists to help estimate hearing threshold and to aid in differential diagnosis

Bone Conduction (BC): method of testing with a bone conduction oscillator such that the signal bypasses the outer and middle ears and delivers to the inner ear and central auditory nervous system

Calibration: process by which equipment is measured to make certain that it is adhering to specialized standards

Complex Harmonic Motion: complex sounds that combine simple harmonic motions and represent intensity as a function of frequency

Conditioned Play Audiometry: audiometric technique utilized with small children, most often of preschool developmental age, where the child responds by game-playing (throwing a block into a box or placing a ring on a peg) upon hearing a stimulus

Conductive Hearing Loss: type of hearing impairment where the disorder lies in the outer and/or middle ear

Configuration of Hearing Loss: parameter used in audiogram interpretation to determine shape of the audiogram and severity as a function of test frequency

Conventional Audiometric Techniques: most often referring to threshold obtaining procedures where the patient is cognitively able to raise a hand or push a button upon hearing the stimulus

Decibel (dB): measurement of intensity of sound

Frequency: parameter of sound, measured in cycles per second, differences of which are perceived by the listener as changes in pitch

Hertz (Hz): measurement of sound frequency, in cycles per second

Hughson-Westlake Procedure: common procedure for obtaining threshold; the audiologist decreases stimulus intensity by 10 dB with a (+) response and increases by 5 dB with a (−) response

Immittance Audiometry: battery of objective measures to assess middle ear function, as well as integrity of contralateral and ipsilateral acoustic reflex arc

Intensity: parameter of sound, measured in decibels, differences of which are perceived by the listener as changes in loudness

Interaural Attenuation: refers to level at which stimulus intended for the test ear crosses over and is perceived by the nontest ear

Magnitude of Hearing Loss: parameter used in audiogram interpretation to help determine severity of hearing impairment, if any

Masking: procedure whereby the audiologist delivers a noise stimulus to the nontest ear to prevent it from participating in the testing session, so that accurate results may be obtained in the test ear

Maximum Effective Masking: highest intensity level of masking noise theoretically presented to nontest ear that will allow the clinician to obtain accurate thresholds in the test ear without overmasking

Minimum Effective Masking: lowest intensity level of masking noise theoretically presented to nontest ear that will allow the clinician to obtain accurate thresholds in the test ear without undermasking

Mixed Hearing Loss: type of hearing impairment where the disorder lies within the conductive and the sensorineural mechanisms

Otoacoustic Emissions (OAEs): physiologic measure correlating with outer hair cell function of the cochlea, utilized by the audiologist to help estimate hearing threshold and to assist in differential diagnosis

Overmasking: during clinical masking, this term refers to an inaccurately high intensity level of noise presented to the nontest ear, such that the noise crosses over to the test ear and interferes with obtaining true thresholds

Phase: parameter of sound that describes its temporal aspects and/or temporal relationships among sounds

Plateau: a clinical masking term referring to a range of noise at which effective masking occurs and true thresholds may be obtained

Sensorineural Hearing Loss: type of hearing impairment where the disorder lies in the inner ear and/or VIIIth nerve

Simple Harmonic Motion (SHM): simplest form of sound, represented by a sinusoidal waveform, showing frequency along the abscissa and intensity along the ordinate

Sound Pressure Level Meter (SPLM): piece of laboratory equipment used to measure sound intensity in dB Sound Pressure Level

Symmetry of Hearing Loss: parameter used in audiogram interpretation to compare sensitivity in one ear to that of the other ear

Three-Frequency Pure-Tone Average (PTA): average of thresholds at 500, 1000, and 2000 Hz in the same ear. This measure should correlate with the speech threshold and configuration warrants whether a two- or a three-frequency PTA is calculated.

Threshold: the softest intensity level at which a stimulus is heard, at least 50% of the time

Transducer: piece of audiometric equipment that transforms one form of energy to another and is utilized to deliver stimuli to the patient

Two-Frequency Pure-Tone Average (PTA): average of two best frequencies (500, 1000, and/or 2000 Hz) in the same ear. This measure should correlate with the speech threshold and configuration warrants whether a two- or a three-frequency PTA is calculated.

Tympanogram: objective measure that helps to assess middle ear function, particularly in terms of pressure and compliance

Type of Hearing Loss: parameter used in audiogram interpretation to help determine anatomic site of disorder

Undermasking: during clinical masking, this term refers to an inaccurately low intensity level of noise presented to the nontest ear, such that the tone still crosses over (to the nontest ear) and interferes with obtaining of true thresholds in the test ear

Visual Reinforcement Audiometry (VRA): technique utilized for ascertaining threshold with pediatric patients, whereby the child lateralizes to a lighted toy whenever the stimulus is heard

Index

A

ABG (air-bone gaps)
  and BC thresholds, 95
  definition of significant,
    72–73, 95, 205
  documenting on audiograms,
    54
  and initial noise intensity
    level to present, 150
  and overmasking potential,
    113
  and threshold shift, 102
ABLB (alternate binaural
    loudness balancing), 199
ABR (auditory brainstem
    response), 200, 210
  and acoustic reflex delay,
    185, 187
  and childhood testing, 147,
    152
  and diagnostic information,
    114
  and differential diagnosis, 189
  hearing screening, 147, 152
  newborn/infant screening,
    118

and nonorganic hearing loss,
    132, 138
AC (air-conduction)
  and air-bone gaps (ABG), 54
  audiometric symbols, 51, 53,
    54
  versus BC (bone conduction)
    signals, 29, 30
  and BC threshold results, 62
  crossover by
    at 500 Hz, 93
  diagnosis with other than
    pure-tone audiometry, 97
  and magnitude
    determination, 70
  masking
    microphones, 97–98
    plateau determination,
      97–102
    process/procedure,
      105–107
    results recording, 108–109
    during testing, 88–89
  SAL (sensorineural acuity
    level) testing, 110–112
  testing/process, 26–27
  threshold testing, 56–59